New Approaches to Wellbeing

How Innovative Techniques, Holistic Strategies, and Cutting-Edge Research Shape the Future of Wellness

Harper Faith

ISBN: 978-1-77961-999-0
Imprint: Play Far Away
Copyright © 2024 Harper Faith.
All Rights Reserved.

Contents

Introduction: Understanding Mental Health and Wellbeing   1
    The Importance of Mental Health   1
    Contemporary Approaches to Mental Health and Wellbeing   13

Innovative Techniques in Mental Health and Wellbeing   23
    Cognitive Behavioral Therapy   23
    Mindfulness-Based Interventions   29
    Art Therapy   39
    Yoga and Meditation   48
    Expressive Writing   57

Holistic Strategies for Mental Health and Wellbeing   65
    Nutrition and Mental Health   65
    Exercise and Physical Activity   73
    Sleep and Mental Wellness   83
    Social Support and Connection   92
    Self-Care Practices   101

Cutting-Edge Research in Mental Health and Wellbeing   111
    Advancements in Neuroscience and Mental Health   111
    Innovative Technologies in Mental Health Care   120
    Psychedelic-Assisted Therapy   131
    Epigenetics and Mental Health   138
    Cultural Considerations in Mental Health Research   148

The Future of Mental Health and Wellbeing   157
    Challenges and Opportunities for Mental Health Care   157
    Emerging Trends in Mental Health Research and Practice   165
    A Call for Action: Advocacy and Policy in Mental Health   175

Conclusion: Shaping a Transformed Mental Health Landscape 184

Index 193

Introduction: Understanding Mental Health and Wellbeing

The Importance of Mental Health

Definition and Scope of Mental Health

Mental health refers to a person's emotional, psychological, and social well-being. It affects how individuals think, feel, and act, and also influences their ability to handle stress, relate to others, and make choices that promote their overall well-being. Mental health is not just the absence of mental illness; it encompasses the positive aspects of mental well-being, such as resilience, self-esteem, and the ability to navigate life's challenges.

The scope of mental health is broad and encompasses various aspects of human life. It includes the promotion of mental well-being, prevention of mental disorders, and the treatment and rehabilitation of individuals who have a diagnosed mental illness. Mental health is not limited to any specific age group, gender, or socioeconomic background; it affects people across all walks of life.

In understanding the scope of mental health, it is essential to recognize that it is a multidimensional concept. The World Health Organization (WHO) defines mental health as "a state of well-being in which every individual realizes their own potential, can cope with the normal stresses of life, can work productively and fruitfully, and is able to make a contribution to their community."

Mental health is influenced by various individual, social, and environmental factors. These factors include biological factors (such as genetics and brain chemistry), life experiences (such as trauma or abuse), family history of mental health problems, and ongoing physical health conditions. Additionally, social determinants of mental health, such as poverty, discrimination, and access to healthcare, also play a significant role in shaping mental well-being.

The understanding of mental health has evolved over time. Historically, mental health was often stigmatized, and individuals with mental health conditions were subjected to social exclusion and discrimination. However, modern perspectives on mental health emphasize the importance of destigmatization and prioritizing mental well-being as a fundamental aspect of overall health.

It is crucial to recognize the interplay between mental health and physical health. Mental health conditions can have a significant impact on physical health outcomes, and vice versa. For example, individuals with chronic physical conditions, such as diabetes or cardiovascular disease, may be at a higher risk for mental health disorders. Similarly, individuals with mental health conditions may experience a range of physical health problems, including increased risk for chronic diseases and compromised immune function.

The scope of mental health also extends beyond the individual level and encompasses community and societal factors. Mental health promotion involves creating supportive environments, fostering social connections, and implementing policies that prioritize mental well-being. It requires collaboration across various sectors, including education, healthcare, workplaces, and community organizations.

Mental health is a dynamic and ever-evolving field that continues to be shaped by research, innovation, and advancements in various disciplines. As our understanding of mental health deepens, so does our ability to develop effective interventions, therapies, and strategies to promote mental well-being and address mental health disorders.

To gain a comprehensive understanding of mental health, it is important to explore the different perspectives and approaches that contribute to its definition and scope. This includes recognizing the influence of cultural, social, and contextual factors on mental health and well-being. Mental health is a complex and intricate field, and its study requires an interdisciplinary approach that integrates knowledge from psychology, neuroscience, sociology, anthropology, and other related disciplines.

Overall, mental health encompasses the emotional, psychological, and social well-being of individuals, and understanding its definition and scope is essential for promoting positive mental well-being and addressing mental health issues effectively. It calls for a holistic and multidimensional approach that recognizes the interconnectedness between mental and physical health, as well as the importance of sociocultural factors in shaping mental well-being. By expanding our knowledge and promoting mental health awareness, we can work towards creating a more compassionate and supportive society that prioritizes the mental well-being of all its members.

Historical Perspectives on Mental Health

Throughout history, the understanding and treatment of mental health have evolved significantly. The historical perspectives on mental health provide insight into how societies have perceived and responded to mental health issues. This section explores key milestones and shifts in thinking that have shaped our current understanding of mental health.

Ancient Beliefs and Supernatural Explanations

In ancient times, mental health disorders were often attributed to supernatural causes and spiritual beliefs. Ancient civilizations, such as the Egyptians, Greeks, and Romans, believed that mental illnesses were punishments from the gods or resulted from demonic possession. Shamanism and exorcism were common methods used to expel evil spirits or restore a balance between individuals and the spiritual realm.

These supernatural explanations limited the understanding of mental health and led to stigmatization and mistreatment of individuals with mental disorders. It was not until the emergence of early philosophical and medical traditions that a shift towards more rational perspectives began.

Greek and Roman Contributions

The ancient Greeks and Romans made significant contributions to the understanding of mental health. Influential Greek physicians, including Hippocrates and Galen, rejected supernatural explanations and proposed a more naturalistic approach.

Hippocrates, often referred to as the father of medicine, proposed the theory of the "Four Humors." According to this theory, an imbalance of bodily fluids (blood, phlegm, yellow bile, and black bile) caused mental disorders. Treatment involved restoring the balance through methods such as diet, exercise, and purging.

The Roman physician Galen expanded on Hippocrates' theories and emphasized the importance of psychological and environmental factors in mental health. His approach foreshadowed the biopsychosocial model, which recognizes the interplay between biology, psychology, and social factors in mental well-being.

Middle Ages and Renaissance

During the Middle Ages, mental health took a dark turn as society's understanding regressed. Mental disorders were often seen as manifestations of evil or witchcraft, leading to the persecution and brutal treatment of individuals. The mentally ill were subjected to exorcism, torture, and confinement in asylums.

The Renaissance period marked a shift towards more humane treatment approaches and a greater focus on individual experiences. The development of humanism led to a renewed interest in understanding the human mind and behavior. Figures like Paracelsus, a Swiss physician, emphasized the importance of understanding the individual's unique psychological and physiological makeup.

Emergence of Psychiatry and the Medical Model

The 18th and 19th centuries saw the establishment of psychiatry as a medical specialty and the emergence of the medical model for mental health. This model viewed mental illnesses as diseases of the brain, emphasizing the biological origins of mental disorders.

Franz Mesmer, an Austrian physician, introduced mesmerism (later called hypnosis) as a treatment for mental illnesses. Mesmer believed that an imbalance of magnetic fluids in the body caused psychological disorders. Although mesmerism was based on flawed theories, it contributed to the recognition of the mind-body connection in mental health.

The late 19th century witnessed significant advancements in psychiatric understanding, with figures like Emil Kraepelin classifying mental disorders and establishing diagnostic criteria. This laid the foundation for modern psychiatric diagnosis and classification systems.

Psychodynamic and Humanistic Perspectives

The early 20th century brought about new perspectives that shifted the focus from biological explanations to psychodynamic and humanistic approaches. Sigmund Freud, the father of psychoanalysis, emphasized the role of unconscious conflicts and early childhood experiences in shaping mental health. Freud's theories and techniques had a profound impact and paved the way for therapy focused on introspection and insight.

The humanistic perspective, championed by Carl Rogers and Abraham Maslow, emphasized the importance of self-actualization and personal growth in mental well-being. It highlighted the inherent worth and dignity of individuals while focusing on promoting self-awareness and self-acceptance.

Deinstitutionalization and Community Mental Health

The mid-20th century witnessed a paradigm shift from long-term institutionalization to community-based mental health care. Deinstitutionalization aimed to provide treatment and support for individuals with mental illness within their communities. This movement recognized the detrimental effects of institutionalization and aimed to promote integration and recovery.

However, the deinstitutionalization process faced challenges such as the lack of community resources, inadequate funding, and the rise of homelessness among individuals with mental health issues. This highlighted the need for comprehensive community mental health services and support systems.

Current Perspectives and the Biopsychosocial Approach

In recent years, there has been a growing recognition of the complex interplay between biological, psychological, and social factors in mental health. The biopsychosocial model has gained prominence, highlighting the need to consider the biological, psychological, and social determinants of mental well-being.

Contemporary approaches also emphasize the importance of cultural context, social justice, and the destigmatization of mental health. Efforts are being made to address disparities in mental health care and improve access to quality services for diverse populations.

Overall, the historical perspectives on mental health have shaped our understanding and approach to mental well-being. From supernatural beliefs to a biopsychosocial framework, our evolving understanding continues to inform research, treatment, and advocacy efforts in the field of mental health. By learning from the past, we can strive to create a more inclusive, compassionate, and effective system of mental health care.

The Role of Mental Health in Overall Wellbeing

Mental health plays a crucial role in overall wellbeing, encompassing various aspects of our lives, including physical health, relationships, productivity, and personal fulfillment. Understanding the connection between mental health and overall wellbeing is essential for promoting a holistic approach to wellness. In this section, we will explore how mental health influences different dimensions of our lives and the impact it has on our overall wellbeing.

The Interplay between Mental Health and Physical Health

Mental health and physical health are deeply intertwined, with each influencing the other in profound ways. Numerous studies have shown the impact of mental health on physical health outcomes, such as cardiovascular health, immune function, and longevity.

1. Mental Health and Cardiovascular Health: Psychological stress, anxiety, and depression can contribute to the development and progression of cardiovascular diseases, such as hypertension and coronary artery disease. Chronic stress activates the sympathetic nervous system, leading to increased heart rate and blood pressure, which, over time, can negatively impact cardiovascular health.

2. Mental Health and Immune Function: Psychological distress and negative emotions can suppress immune function, making individuals more susceptible to infections and impairing their ability to recover from illness. Chronic stress, for instance, can affect immune system regulation and increase inflammation, which is implicated in various chronic diseases.

3. Mental Health and Longevity: Poor mental health, including conditions like depression and chronic stress, has been associated with increased mortality rates. The negative effects of mental health on physical health can contribute to a shorter lifespan and reduced quality of life.

It is important, therefore, to address mental health concerns to promote better physical health outcomes and overall wellbeing.

The Influence of Mental Health on Relationships and Social Wellbeing

Mental health significantly impacts our relationships and social interactions, playing a vital role in our ability to connect with others, form meaningful relationships, and experience a sense of belonging. Here are some key aspects of the role of mental health in relationships and social wellbeing:

1. Emotional Wellbeing: Mental health influences our emotional state, including our ability to manage and regulate emotions. Individuals with good mental health are more likely to have stable emotional well-being, which can foster healthy and fulfilling relationships.

2. Communication and Empathy: Mental health has a direct impact on our communication skills and ability to empathize with others. Improved mental health can enhance effective communication and enable us to understand and respond to the emotions and needs of those around us.

3. Social Support: Maintaining positive mental health is crucial for accessing and providing social support. People with good mental health are more likely to seek

help when needed and offer support to others, thereby strengthening social bonds and creating a supportive network.

4. Sense of Belonging: Mental health issues, such as anxiety and depression, can lead to feelings of isolation and detachment. Conversely, good mental health fosters a sense of belonging, which is vital for social integration and overall wellbeing.

The Impact of Mental Health on Productivity and Personal Fulfillment

Mental health plays a significant role in our productivity and personal fulfillment, affecting our ability to perform daily tasks, pursue goals, and find meaning and satisfaction in our lives. Some key aspects of the influence of mental health on productivity and personal fulfillment include:

1. Cognitive Functioning: Optimal mental health is associated with improved cognitive abilities, such as concentration, memory, and decision-making. Good mental health supports effective problem-solving skills and enhances productivity in various domains.

2. Work Performance: Mental health problems, such as stress, anxiety, and burnout, can have a detrimental impact on work performance. Addressing mental health concerns and promoting mental well-being in the workplace can lead to higher productivity, job satisfaction, and overall success.

3. Goal Attainment: Mental health influences our motivation, resilience, and ability to set and achieve goals. When mental health is prioritized, individuals are more likely to experience a sense of purpose, discover their strengths, and work towards personal fulfillment.

4. Quality of Life: Mental health is crucial for experiencing a fulfilling and meaningful life. Poor mental health can diminish overall life satisfaction and hinder the ability to engage in activities that bring joy and purpose.

It is evident that mental health is a critical determinant of our overall wellbeing, impacting our physical health, relationships, productivity, and personal fulfillment. By recognizing the multifaceted role of mental health, we can strive towards a holistic approach to wellness that prioritizes mental well-being alongside physical well-being. In the next sections, we will explore innovative techniques and holistic strategies that can further enhance mental health and overall wellbeing.

Stigma and Discrimination Surrounding Mental Health

Stigma and discrimination surrounding mental health are significant barriers that impact individuals seeking help and accessing proper care. These negative attitudes and beliefs are prevalent across societies and contribute to the stigma associated with mental health conditions. Understanding the nature of stigma and discrimination is essential in developing effective strategies to promote mental health and wellbeing.

Definition and Nature of Stigma

Stigma can be defined as a social process in which an individual or group is negatively labeled based on certain characteristics or attributes. In the context of mental health, stigma refers to the stereotypes, prejudices, and discrimination faced by individuals with mental health conditions. Stigma often leads to social exclusion, marginalization, and the denial of basic human rights.

The nature of mental health stigma is complex and multifaceted. It can manifest in several forms, including public stigma, self-stigma, and structural stigma. Public stigma involves societal attitudes and beliefs that lead to the devaluation and marginalization of individuals with mental health conditions. Self-stigma, on the other hand, refers to the internalization of these negative beliefs by people with mental illness, leading to reduced self-esteem and self-efficacy. Structural stigma refers to the discriminatory practices and policies embedded within institutions and systems, limiting access to resources and services for individuals with mental health conditions.

Causes and Influences of Stigma

Stigma towards mental health is influenced by various factors, including cultural, historical, and sociopolitical contexts. In many cultures, mental health conditions are stigmatized due to cultural beliefs, myths, and misconceptions surrounding the causes and nature of mental illness. Historical perspectives have also contributed to the stigma, as mental health has often been misunderstood or associated with supernatural or moral failings.

Sociopolitical factors, including discriminatory policies and lack of resources, perpetuate mental health stigma. The lack of funding and inadequate mental health services reinforce the perception that mental illnesses are less deserving of attention and resources compared to physical health conditions. Media portrayal of mental illness can also play a role in shaping public attitudes and stereotypes.

Impact of Stigma and Discrimination

Stigma and discrimination have pervasive effects on individuals living with mental health conditions. They create significant barriers to seeking help, leading to delayed treatment and exacerbation of symptoms. Individuals may experience feelings of shame, guilt, and isolation, which can negatively impact their mental health and quality of life. Stigmatized individuals are less likely to disclose their condition, leading to social withdrawal and reduced social support networks.

Stigma also affects treatment outcomes and recovery. Negative perceptions and stereotypes can lead to inadequate care, as healthcare professionals may have lower expectations for individuals with mental health conditions, resulting in substandard treatment. Discrimination in employment, education, and housing further limits opportunities and socioeconomic integration for individuals with mental health conditions.

Addressing Stigma and Discrimination

Addressing stigma and discrimination surrounding mental health requires a multifaceted approach involving individuals, communities, organizations, and governments. Education and awareness campaigns play a crucial role in challenging stereotypes, dispelling myths, and promoting understanding and empathy. Such initiatives should focus on promoting positive attitudes, highlighting the prevalence and diversity of mental health conditions, and emphasizing recovery and resilience.

Legislation and policy reforms are necessary to address structural stigma and ensure equal access to mental health services. These reforms should prioritize mental health in healthcare systems, incorporate anti-discrimination laws, and promote inclusivity and diversity in the workforce.

It is essential to involve individuals with lived experience of mental health conditions in designing and implementing strategies to combat stigma. Peer support programs, advocacy groups, and community-based initiatives can empower individuals to challenge stigma, promote acceptance, and provide support to those in need.

Example: Workplace Mental Health

Workplace stigma and discrimination surrounding mental health is a common issue faced by individuals with mental health conditions. Employees may hesitate to disclose their conditions due to fear of negative consequences, such as being treated differently, denied promotions, or even termination. Employers have a responsibility to create a supportive and inclusive work environment.

To address workplace stigma, organizations can implement mental health awareness training for managers and employees, fostering a culture of understanding and empathy. Policies and practices should be developed to protect employees' rights and ensure reasonable accommodations for individuals with mental health conditions. Providing resources such as Employee Assistance

Programs and mental health support services can promote early intervention and timely access to care.

Conclusion

Stigma and discrimination surrounding mental health continue to be significant barriers that hinder the wellbeing and recovery of individuals with mental health conditions. By understanding the nature, causes, and impacts of stigma, we can develop comprehensive approaches to challenge and reduce these barriers. It is crucial to promote awareness, advocate for policy reforms, and create supportive environments that foster inclusivity, acceptance, and equality for everyone, regardless of their mental health status.

The Global Mental Health Crisis

The global mental health crisis is a pressing issue that affects individuals, communities, and societies worldwide. It is characterized by the increasing prevalence of mental health disorders, inadequate access to mental health services, and the stigma and discrimination faced by those with mental illness. This section aims to provide an overview of the current state of the global mental health crisis, its causes and consequences, and potential strategies for addressing and mitigating its impact.

Prevalence of Mental Health Disorders

Mental health disorders, including depression, anxiety, schizophrenia, bipolar disorder, and substance abuse, are prevalent worldwide, affecting people of all ages, genders, and socioeconomic backgrounds. According to the World Health Organization (WHO), approximately 1 in 4 individuals will experience a mental health disorder at some point in their lives. The burden of mental illness is substantial, as it significantly impairs individuals' quality of life, functioning, and productivity.

The prevalence of mental health disorders varies across countries and regions, but there are common risk factors that contribute to their occurrence. These risk factors include biological factors (such as genetics and brain chemistry), environmental factors (such as trauma and exposure to violence), psychological factors (such as stress and trauma), and social determinants of health (such as poverty and social inequality).

Barriers to Accessing Mental Health Services

Despite the high prevalence of mental health disorders, there are significant barriers to accessing appropriate and timely mental health services. These barriers are particularly prevalent in low- and middle-income countries, where mental health resources are often limited and underfunded.

One major barrier is the shortage of mental health professionals, including psychiatrists, psychologists, and social workers, especially in rural and remote areas. This shortage is exacerbated by the brain drain phenomenon, where mental health professionals migrate to high-income countries for better opportunities and higher salaries.

Another barrier to accessing mental health services is the high cost of treatment and medication. Many individuals are unable to afford the necessary care due to financial constraints, lack of insurance coverage, or the absence of mental health services within their communities.

Stigma and discrimination associated with mental illness also serve as significant barriers to seeking help. Many societies hold negative attitudes and beliefs about mental health, leading to the social isolation and marginalization of individuals with mental illness. This stigma prevents individuals from seeking treatment and support, resulting in delayed or inadequate care.

Consequences of the Global Mental Health Crisis

The consequences of the global mental health crisis are far-reaching and impact individuals, families, communities, and economies. On an individual level, untreated mental health disorders can lead to impaired functioning, decreased quality of life, and increased risk of suicide. Mental health issues can also manifest as physical health problems due to the interconnectedness of mental and physical well-being.

At the societal level, the global mental health crisis poses significant economic burdens. The cost of mental health disorders includes direct healthcare costs, productivity losses, and the strain on social support systems. These economic consequences result from decreased productivity in the workplace, increased healthcare expenditures, and the impact on families who shoulder the burden of caregiving.

Furthermore, the global mental health crisis exacerbates existing social inequalities. Research shows that individuals with mental illness are more likely to experience unemployment, poverty, homelessness, and incarceration. This perpetuates a cycle of disadvantage and further marginalizes vulnerable populations.

Strategies for Addressing the Global Mental Health Crisis

Addressing the global mental health crisis requires a comprehensive and multi-faceted approach that encompasses various strategies. Some key strategies for tackling this crisis include:

1. Policy and Advocacy: Governments and international organizations should prioritize mental health in their policy agendas, allocate sufficient resources to mental health services, and work towards reducing stigma and discrimination.

2. Integrated Care: Mental health should be integrated into primary healthcare systems to ensure early identification, diagnosis, and treatment of mental health disorders. Collaborative care models involving multidisciplinary teams can improve access to services and enhance outcomes.

3. Capacity Building and Workforce Development: Efforts should be made to train and retain mental health professionals, especially in underserved areas. This includes establishing training programs, providing financial incentives, and implementing telemedicine initiatives to reach remote communities.

4. Community-Based Interventions: Strengthening community-based mental health services, such as non-governmental organizations and community health workers, can improve access, reduce stigma, and provide culturally appropriate care.

5. Promotion of Mental Wellbeing: Promoting mental wellbeing through public awareness campaigns, education, and prevention programs is crucial. This includes teaching coping skills, stress management techniques, and promoting healthy lifestyles.

6. Global Collaboration: International collaboration is essential for sharing best practices, research, and resources. This includes partnerships between governments, non-governmental organizations, and academia to address the global mental health crisis collectively.

It is important to recognize that addressing the global mental health crisis is a complex and ongoing process. It requires sustained commitment, collaboration, and innovation to ensure that mental health and wellbeing are prioritized and accessible for all individuals, regardless of their geographical location or socioeconomic status.

Conclusion

The global mental health crisis represents a significant challenge for individuals, communities, and societies worldwide. The high prevalence of mental health disorders, coupled with barriers to accessing care and the consequences of untreated mental illness, demands urgent attention and action.

By implementing comprehensive strategies that address the root causes of mental health disorders, promote access to services, and reduce stigma, it is possible to transform the global mental health landscape. This transformation requires a collaborative effort, involving policymakers, healthcare professionals, communities, and individuals themselves.

Through concerted efforts, the journey towards a world where mental health is prioritized, and individuals can live fulfilling lives with optimal wellbeing is attainable. The global mental health crisis can be addressed, and the future of mental health can be shaped to ensure better outcomes for all.

Contemporary Approaches to Mental Health and Wellbeing

Traditional Biomedical Model

In the field of mental health, the traditional biomedical model has long been the dominant approach to understanding and treating mental health disorders. This model views mental illnesses as purely biological in nature, with the focus primarily on identifying and treating specific physiological abnormalities or imbalances in the brain.

Under the traditional biomedical model, mental health disorders are often attributed to chemical imbalances in the brain, genetic factors, or abnormalities in brain structure and function. Treatment approaches typically rely heavily on the use of medications, such as antidepressants, antipsychotics, or mood stabilizers, to target specific symptoms and alleviate the underlying biological causes.

While the traditional biomedical model has made significant advancements in the diagnosis and treatment of mental health disorders, it has its limitations. It tends to oversimplify the complex and multifaceted nature of mental health and overlooks the impact of psychological, social, and environmental factors on an individual's mental wellbeing.

One of the main criticisms of the traditional biomedical model is its overemphasis on pharmacological interventions. While medications can be effective in managing symptoms, they often do not address the underlying causes of mental health disorders. Additionally, the reliance on medications can lead to a reductionist approach, where mental health conditions are solely viewed as chemical imbalances to be corrected through medication.

Another limitation of the traditional biomedical model is its failure to take into account the subjective experiences and lived realities of individuals with mental health disorders. It tends to pathologize distressing thoughts, emotions, and behaviors without considering their context or meaning. This can perpetuate stigma and hinder a person's journey towards recovery and wellbeing.

It is crucial to recognize that mental health disorders are influenced by a range of factors, including biological, psychological, social, and cultural factors. The traditional biomedical model often neglects the importance of psychological and social interventions in promoting mental health and wellbeing.

However, it is important to note that the traditional biomedical model has played a significant role in advancing our understanding of mental health and developing effective treatments. Medications have been lifesaving for many individuals and have provided significant relief from symptoms of mental health disorders.

Moving forward, there is a growing recognition of the need for a more holistic and integrative approach to mental health. This includes considering the individual's unique psychological and social circumstances, as well as addressing the underlying causes and promoting overall wellbeing.

While the traditional biomedical model continues to be an important component of mental health care, it should be complemented by other approaches that take into account the complexity of mental health and the interplay of biological, psychological, social, and environmental factors. This involves incorporating evidence-based practices from various therapeutic modalities, such as cognitive behavioral therapy, mindfulness-based interventions, and art therapy, to provide comprehensive and person-centered care.

By adopting a more integrative and holistic approach, mental health professionals can better support individuals in their journey towards recovery and overall wellbeing. This involves recognizing the importance of individualized treatment plans, addressing the broader social determinants of mental health, and fostering collaboration and interdisciplinary approaches in the field of mental health care.

In conclusion, while the traditional biomedical model has made significant contributions to our understanding and treatment of mental health disorders, it is essential to move towards a more holistic and person-centered approach. Integrating psychological, social, and environmental interventions along with biological treatments can help shape the future of mental health and wellbeing by providing more comprehensive and effective care for individuals living with mental health disorders.

The Shift towards Holistic Approaches

In recent years, there has been a significant shift in the field of mental health towards holistic approaches. This shift recognizes the interconnectedness of various aspects of an individual's life and well-being, and the need to address these different dimensions in order to promote overall mental health. Holistic approaches take into consideration not only the physiological and psychological factors that contribute to mental health, but also social, cultural, and spiritual aspects.

One of the key principles of holistic approaches is the recognition that mental health cannot be separated from physical health. The mind and body are closely intertwined, and any disturbances in one can have an impact on the other. Therefore, holistic approaches emphasize the importance of maintaining a healthy lifestyle that includes regular exercise, proper nutrition, and adequate sleep. These factors play a crucial role in supporting mental well-being and resilience.

Moreover, holistic approaches consider the role of social and cultural factors in shaping mental health. Social support and connectedness have been shown to be protective factors against mental health problems. Being a part of a supportive community or having strong relationships can provide individuals with a sense of belonging and reduce feelings of loneliness and isolation. Cultural factors, such as values, beliefs, and practices, also contribute to mental health outcomes. Holistic approaches recognize the importance of cultural competence in mental health care, and the need to address cultural differences and provide culturally appropriate interventions.

Another important aspect of holistic approaches is the recognition of the spiritual dimension of mental health. While spirituality is often associated with religious beliefs, it can also encompass a broader sense of meaning, purpose, and connection to something greater than oneself. Spiritual practices, such as meditation, mindfulness, or engaging in meaningful activities, can enhance mental well-being by promoting inner peace, resilience, and a sense of purpose.

Holistic approaches also emphasize the need to address the underlying causes of mental health problems, rather than just focusing on symptom management. This involves taking a person-centered approach that considers the individual's unique circumstances, experiences, and preferences. By understanding the individual's context and life circumstances, holistic approaches can identify and address the root causes of mental health issues, and provide interventions that are tailored to meet the individual's specific needs.

To effectively implement holistic approaches in mental health care, collaboration and integration across different disciplines and sectors is essential. This includes engaging professionals from various backgrounds, such as psychologists, psychiatrists, social workers, nutritionists, and alternative therapists. By working together, these professionals can provide a comprehensive and multi-faceted approach to mental health care that addresses the diverse needs of individuals.

In conclusion, the shift towards holistic approaches in mental health recognizes that mental well-being is influenced by various factors, including physical, social, cultural, and spiritual dimensions. Addressing these different aspects is crucial for promoting overall mental health and well-being. Holistic approaches emphasize the connection between mind and body, the importance of social support and cultural competence, and the need to address the underlying causes of mental health problems. By adopting a holistic approach, mental health care can become more comprehensive and person-centered, leading to improved outcomes for individuals.

Integrative Approaches to Mental Health and Wellbeing

In recent years, there has been a significant shift in the approach to mental health and wellbeing. Traditional biomedical models, which focus mainly on pharmacological interventions and symptom management, are being supplemented and, in some cases, replaced by integrative approaches. Integrative approaches prioritize the holistic understanding of individuals and strive to address the multiple interconnected factors that contribute to mental health and wellbeing.

The Biopsychosocial Model

One key concept underpinning integrative approaches is the biopsychosocial model. This model recognizes that mental health and wellbeing are influenced by a combination of biological, psychological, and social factors. It emphasizes the interconnectedness of these factors and how they interact to impact an individual's mental health.

The biological aspect of the biopsychosocial model acknowledges the role of genetics, brain chemistry, and the physical body in mental health. It highlights the importance of understanding how biological factors can contribute to mental health disorders and informs targeted interventions, such as medication or nutritional interventions.

The psychological aspect of the model focuses on the individual's thoughts, emotions, and behaviors. It recognizes the significance of psychological factors, such as cognitive patterns, trauma history, and coping mechanisms, in the development and maintenance of mental health conditions. Psychological interventions, such as cognitive-behavioral therapy (CBT) and mindfulness-based interventions, are commonly used within integrative approaches.

The social aspect of the biopsychosocial model highlights the influence of social and environmental factors on mental health. It acknowledges the impact of socio-economic status, cultural norms, family dynamics, and social support networks on mental wellbeing. Integrative approaches consider the importance of creating supportive social environments and promoting positive social connections.

Integrating Different Modalities

Integrative approaches to mental health and wellbeing aim to combine different therapeutic modalities and treatments to address the complex and multifaceted nature of mental health conditions. By integrating various approaches, practitioners can provide a more comprehensive and personalized approach to each individual's unique needs.

For example, a person experiencing anxiety may benefit from a combination of cognitive-behavioral therapy, yoga, and nutritional interventions. The cognitive-behavioral therapy component can help identify and challenge maladaptive thought patterns, while yoga can provide relaxation techniques and promote mind-body awareness. Nutritional interventions can address potential deficiencies or imbalances that may contribute to anxiety symptoms.

Integrative approaches also recognize the importance of tailoring treatment plans to individual needs and preferences. What works for one person may not work for another, and it is essential to consider the individual's values, cultural background, and personal goals in the treatment process. This personalized approach helps enhance engagement and motivation, leading to better outcomes.

Collaborative Care

Another crucial aspect of integrative approaches to mental health and wellbeing is collaborative care. Collaborative care involves a coordinated effort among different healthcare providers, such as psychiatrists, psychologists, social workers, and other specialists, to ensure comprehensive and holistic support for individuals with mental health conditions.

By working together, healthcare providers can share expertise, integrate different treatment approaches, and tailor interventions to the individual's needs. Collaborative care also involves active involvement from the individual receiving treatment, their family members, and the wider community to create a supportive network.

An example of collaborative care could involve a person with depression receiving input from a psychiatrist, therapist, and nutritionist. The psychiatrist may prescribe medication to address the biological aspect of depression, while the therapist provides psychotherapy to help the individual process emotions and develop coping skills. The nutritionist can offer guidance on dietary changes that may support improved mood and overall wellbeing.

Evaluating the Effectiveness of Integrative Approaches

Assessing the effectiveness of integrative approaches to mental health and wellbeing is crucial for evidence-informed practice. It involves conducting rigorous research studies to determine the impact of these approaches on various mental health conditions.

Researchers employ various methods to evaluate integrative approaches, such as randomized controlled trials, qualitative research, and systematic reviews. These studies aim to measure outcomes related to symptom reduction, quality of life, functional improvement, and overall wellbeing.

It is important to acknowledge the challenges in evaluating integrative approaches, given the complexity and individualized nature of treatments. However, ongoing research and evaluation are pivotal in shaping the future of integrative mental health care.

An Unconventional Example: Animal-Assisted Therapy

An unconventional yet relevant integrative approach to mental health and wellbeing is animal-assisted therapy. This approach involves incorporating animals, such as dogs or horses, into therapeutic interventions to promote emotional and psychological healing.

Animal-assisted therapy has been shown to improve symptoms of anxiety, depression, and post-traumatic stress disorder (PTSD). Interacting with animals can reduce stress, increase social interaction, and provide a sense of companionship and comfort.

For example, a person with PTSD may engage in equine-assisted therapy, where they interact with horses and participate in various activities, such as grooming or riding. This interaction can help foster trust, build emotional regulation skills, and provide opportunities for processing traumatic experiences.

Although animal-assisted therapy may not be suitable for everyone or for all mental health conditions, it serves as an illustrative example of how unconventional modalities can complement traditional approaches within integrative mental health care.

Key Takeaways

- Integrative approaches to mental health and wellbeing prioritize a holistic understanding of individuals, incorporating biological, psychological, and social factors. - The biopsychosocial model provides a framework for understanding the interconnectedness of these factors in mental health. - Integrative approaches aim to combine different modalities to create personalized and comprehensive treatment plans. - Collaborative care involves coordination among healthcare providers and active involvement from individuals, family members, and the wider community. - Evaluating the effectiveness of integrative approaches requires rigorous research and measurement of outcomes. - Unconventional approaches, such as animal-assisted therapy, can complement traditional modalities within integrative mental health care.

The Role of Culture and Context in Shaping Approaches

Culture and context play a significant role in shaping approaches to mental health and wellbeing. Different cultures have diverse beliefs, values, and practices related to mental health, which greatly influence the understanding and treatment of mental disorders. Additionally, the social, economic, and environmental contexts in which individuals live affect their experiences of mental health and the availability and accessibility of resources for support and treatment.

Cultural Perspectives on Mental Health

Culture influences the perception, expression, and interpretation of mental health and illness. Cultural perspectives shape the understanding of mental health conditions, the attribution of symptoms, and the appropriate interventions for treatment. By considering cultural beliefs and practices, mental health professionals can develop more culturally sensitive and effective approaches to care.

For example, in some cultures, mental health problems may be attributed to supernatural causes, such as witchcraft or demonic possession. Treating these conditions may involve traditional healers, rituals, or spiritual interventions. In contrast, other cultures may emphasize the biomedical model, viewing mental disorders as primarily biological or neurochemical in nature. These cultural variations impact help-seeking behaviors, treatment adherence, and overall mental health outcomes.

Cultural Competence in Mental Health Care

To provide effective mental health care, professionals must possess cultural competence – the ability to understand and address the unique cultural backgrounds and needs of their clients. Cultural competence involves knowledge of cultural practices, values, and beliefs related to mental health, as well as the ability to adapt interventions accordingly.

Cultural competence also requires awareness of one's own cultural biases and assumptions, as well as the impact of power imbalances and systemic injustices on mental health disparities. Recognizing and respecting cultural diversity fosters trust and strengthens therapeutic alliances between mental health providers and individuals seeking care.

Intersectionality and Mental Health

Intersectionality, a concept originating from feminist and critical race theories, highlights the interconnectedness of social identities and the ways in which multiple forms of oppression, such as racism, sexism, homophobia, and ableism, intersect and contribute to health disparities, including mental health.

Understanding the intersectionality of identities is crucial in mental health care to recognize and address the unique challenges faced by individuals who belong to multiple marginalized groups. For example, LGBTQ+ individuals may experience higher rates of mental health issues due to the stress of discrimination and stigma. By considering the intersectionality of identities, mental health professionals can provide more comprehensive and appropriate care.

Incorporating Cultural Considerations in Research and Intervention Development

Cultural considerations are vital in both research and intervention development within the field of mental health. Culturally sensitive research acknowledges the influence of cultural factors on mental health outcomes and seeks to understand how cultural beliefs, practices, and experiences interact with mental health conditions.

Interventions that are culturally adapted and tailored to specific populations have shown to be more effective. This includes incorporating culturally relevant language, symbols, and metaphors into therapy, as well as involving community members and cultural experts in the development and evaluation of interventions.

Challenges and Limitations

Addressing culture and context in mental health care also presents its challenges and limitations. It may be difficult to navigate the complexities of diverse cultural beliefs and practices, especially in multicultural societies. Mental health professionals must strike a balance between respecting cultural traditions and ensuring that interventions are evidence-based and ethically sound. Over-emphasizing cultural differences may reinforce stereotypes or perpetuate harmful practices.

Furthermore, within a particular cultural group, there can be significant variations in beliefs and practices related to mental health. It is essential to avoid generalizations and instead approach each individual with cultural humility, recognizing their unique experiences and perspectives.

Promoting Cultural Competence and Contextual Understanding

To promote cultural competence and understanding of context, mental health training programs and professional organizations should incorporate cultural competence training into curricula and provide ongoing education and supervision. This training should emphasize the importance of self-reflection, awareness of biases, and an empathetic and inclusive approach to care.

Collaboration between mental health professionals and community organizations is also crucial. This partnership can foster community-engaged research, the development of culturally sensitive interventions, and the provision of accessible mental health services that address the specific needs of diverse populations.

Conclusion

Cultural and contextual factors significantly influence approaches to mental health and wellbeing. By recognizing the role of culture and context, mental health professionals can develop more culturally sensitive, inclusive, and effective strategies and interventions. Through ongoing research, training, and collaboration with communities, we can strive for a mental health landscape that embraces the diverse needs and experiences of individuals, promoting holistic wellbeing for all.

Innovative Techniques in Mental Health and Wellbeing

Cognitive Behavioral Therapy

Overview of Cognitive Behavioral Therapy

Cognitive Behavioral Therapy (CBT) is a widely recognized and extensively researched form of psychotherapy that has shown effectiveness in treating a variety of mental health conditions. It is based on the premise that our thoughts, emotions, and behaviors are interconnected, and by identifying and changing negative patterns of thinking and behaving, individuals can improve their mental health and well-being.

CBT is rooted in two main theoretical frameworks: cognitive therapy and behavioral therapy. Cognitive therapy focuses on examining and challenging the irrational and negative thoughts that contribute to distressing emotions and maladaptive behavior. It aims to help individuals develop healthier and more rational ways of thinking. On the other hand, behavioral therapy focuses on the relationship between our actions and our emotions. It emphasizes the importance of identifying and modifying maladaptive behaviors through behavioral experiments and graded exposure.

The core principles of CBT involve a collaborative therapeutic relationship between the therapist and the client, an emphasis on active participation and engagement, and a focus on the here and now. CBT is typically short-term, goal-oriented, and structured, with sessions typically lasting between 45 and 60 minutes.

The process of CBT begins with a thorough assessment of the client's presenting issues and the formulation of an individualized treatment plan. The therapist and client work together to identify the specific thoughts, emotions, and behaviors that contribute to the client's difficulties. Through various techniques and strategies, the therapist helps the client challenge and reframe their negative thoughts, develop alternative, more adaptive beliefs, and practice new coping skills.

One of the key techniques used in CBT is cognitive restructuring, which involves identifying automatic negative thoughts (ANTs) and replacing them with more realistic and positive thoughts. This process helps individuals gain a more balanced perspective and reduce their emotional distress. Cognitive restructuring can be done through various methods such as Socratic questioning, thought records, and cognitive diaries.

Behavioral experiments are another important component of CBT. These experiments involve testing the validity of an individual's negative beliefs by engaging in real-life activities or situations that challenge those beliefs. By gathering evidence that contradicts their negative thoughts, individuals can learn to develop more accurate and adaptive beliefs.

In addition to cognitive restructuring and behavioral experiments, CBT employs a range of other techniques, including relaxation training, psychoeducation, social skills training, problem-solving, and exposure therapy. Each technique is tailored to the unique needs and goals of the client.

CBT has been extensively researched and has demonstrated efficacy in treating a wide range of mental health conditions, including depression, anxiety disorders, eating disorders, substance use disorders, and post-traumatic stress disorder (PTSD). It has also been adapted for use in diverse populations, such as children, adolescents, couples, and older adults.

While CBT has shown strong empirical support, it is important to acknowledge its limitations. CBT may not be suitable for everyone, and some individuals may benefit from alternative or complementary approaches. Additionally, the effectiveness of CBT can vary depending on factors such as the client's motivation and commitment, the therapist's skill and experience, and the presence of co-occurring conditions.

It is worth noting that CBT is not a one-size-fits-all approach, and therapists are encouraged to adapt and integrate various techniques based on the client's specific needs and preferences. Moreover, CBT is often combined with other treatment modalities, such as medication management, to provide a comprehensive and holistic approach to mental health care.

In conclusion, Cognitive Behavioral Therapy (CBT) is a widely recognized and evidence-based form of psychotherapy that aims to help individuals identify and change negative patterns of thinking and behaving. By challenging irrational thoughts and engaging in new behaviors, individuals can improve their mental health and overall well-being. CBT is a collaborative and structured approach that has shown efficacy in treating various mental health conditions. While it has its limitations, CBT continues to be a valuable tool in the field of mental health and is likely to remain a cornerstone in the future of mental health care.

Application of Cognitive Behavioral Therapy in Various Mental Health Disorders

Cognitive Behavioral Therapy (CBT) is a widely recognized and effective approach in the field of mental health. It is based on the principle that our thoughts, feelings, and behaviors are interconnected and influence each other. By identifying and modifying negative thoughts and maladaptive behaviors, CBT aims to improve mental health and overall well-being. In this section, we will explore the application of CBT in various mental health disorders.

Depression

Depression is a common mental health disorder characterized by persistent sadness, loss of interest or pleasure, changes in appetite or sleep patterns, feelings of guilt or worthlessness, and difficulty concentrating. CBT has been extensively studied and proven effective in treating depression.

CBT interventions for depression focus on identifying negative thinking patterns, such as cognitive distortions (e.g., black-and-white thinking, overgeneralization) and negative self-talk. Through cognitive restructuring techniques, individuals learn to challenge and replace these negative thoughts with more realistic and positive ones. They are also encouraged to engage in activities they previously enjoyed and set achievable goals.

For example, a person with depression may have a cognitive distortion of "all-or-nothing" thinking, where they see situations as either perfect or total failures. In therapy, they may learn to identify this pattern and challenge it by considering alternative outcomes and embracing a more balanced perspective.

Anxiety Disorders

Anxiety disorders encompass a range of conditions characterized by excessive worry, fear, and physiological arousal. Examples include generalized anxiety disorder (GAD), panic disorder, social anxiety disorder, and specific phobias. CBT has shown promising results in the treatment of anxiety disorders.

CBT interventions for anxiety disorders typically involve cognitive restructuring techniques, exposure therapy, and the development of coping strategies. The goal is to help individuals identify and challenge anxious thoughts, gradually confront anxiety-inducing situations, and learn methods to manage the associated physical symptoms.

For instance, a person with social anxiety disorder may have an irrational fear of public speaking. Through exposure therapy, they would gradually be exposed to speaking in public, starting with small and manageable steps. Cognitive techniques, such as challenging negative thoughts about their performance, can also be used to reduce anxiety in such situations.

Obsessive-Compulsive Disorder (OCD)

OCD is a chronic mental health disorder characterized by intrusive thoughts (obsessions) and repetitive behaviors or rituals (compulsions). CBT, particularly a specific form called Exposure and Response Prevention (ERP), is considered the first-line treatment for OCD.

ERP involves gradually exposing individuals to their obsessions, allowing the anxiety to naturally subside without engaging in the associated compulsions. This process helps to disprove the irrational beliefs that underlie the obsessions and break the cycle of anxiety and compulsive behaviors.

For example, a person with OCD may have an obsession related to contamination fears and engage in excessive handwashing as a compulsion. During therapy, the individual would be exposed to situations that trigger their obsession, such as touching a doorknob, and then prevented from engaging in handwashing. Through repeated exposure, they will learn to tolerate the anxiety and realize that their feared consequences do not occur.

Eating Disorders

Eating disorders, including anorexia nervosa, bulimia nervosa, and binge eating disorder, are complex mental health conditions that involve distorted body image, extreme food behaviors, and negative thoughts related to body weight and shape. CBT has shown promising results in the treatment of eating disorders, often in combination with other therapeutic approaches.

CBT interventions for eating disorders focus on underlying cognitive distortions and dysfunctional beliefs regarding body image and food. Techniques such as cognitive restructuring, behavioral experiments, and self-monitoring are used to challenge and modify these thoughts and behaviors.

For instance, a person with an eating disorder may have a cognitive distortion of "emotional reasoning," where they believe their emotions dictate reality (e.g., "I feel fat, so I must be fat"). In therapy, they may be encouraged to question the evidence supporting this belief and explore alternative interpretations. Behavioral experiments, such as challenging body checking behaviors or rigid food rules, can also help individuals test the validity of their beliefs.

Post-Traumatic Stress Disorder (PTSD)

PTSD is a mental health disorder that develops after exposure to a traumatic event. Symptoms include intrusive thoughts or memories, flashbacks, hypervigilance, and avoidance of trauma-related stimuli. CBT, particularly a technique called Cognitive Processing Therapy (CPT), is an evidence-based treatment for PTSD.

CPT focuses on helping individuals identify and change maladaptive thoughts and beliefs related to the traumatic event. The therapy involves examining how the trauma has affected their beliefs about themselves, others, and the world, and developing more adaptive ways of thinking.

For example, a person with PTSD may have a negative core belief, such as "I am permanently damaged" or "The world is dangerous." Through CPT, they would work to challenge these beliefs by exploring evidence that contradicts them and developing more balanced and accurate perspectives.

In conclusion, CBT is a valuable therapeutic approach in the treatment of various mental health disorders. By targeting negative thoughts, beliefs, and behaviors, CBT helps individuals develop healthier thinking patterns, reduce distressing symptoms, and improve their overall well-being. It is important to note that CBT is often used in conjunction with other interventions and tailored to the specific needs of each individual.

Effectiveness and Limitations of Cognitive Behavioral Therapy

Cognitive Behavioral Therapy (CBT) is a widely recognized and effective approach for treating various mental health disorders. It is a form of psychotherapy that focuses on the connection between an individual's thoughts, emotions, and behaviors, and how these interactions can influence mental well-being. CBT aims to identify and change negative or maladaptive thought patterns and behaviors, ultimately improving overall mental health.

Effectiveness of Cognitive Behavioral Therapy

Numerous studies have demonstrated the effectiveness of CBT in treating a range of mental health conditions, including depression, anxiety disorders, post-traumatic stress disorder (PTSD), obsessive-compulsive disorder (OCD), and eating disorders. Research has consistently shown that CBT can lead to significant improvements in symptoms, with outcomes comparable to or even better than medication in some cases.

One key aspect of CBT's effectiveness is its collaborative nature. Therapists and clients work together to identify and modify unhelpful thoughts and behaviors, empowering individuals to take an active role in their treatment. By developing coping skills and strategies, clients can better navigate their daily lives and manage symptoms more effectively.

Furthermore, CBT often provides long-lasting benefits, even after therapy has ended. The skills and techniques learned during CBT sessions can be applied in real-life situations, equipping individuals with tools to maintain their mental well-being beyond therapy.

Limitations of Cognitive Behavioral Therapy

While CBT is an effective treatment modality, it is not without its limitations. It is essential to be aware of these limitations to ensure appropriate treatment planning and to manage expectations.

Firstly, CBT may not be suitable for everyone. Some individuals may struggle with engaging in therapy, particularly if they have difficulty identifying their thoughts and emotions or struggle with self-reflection. Additionally, certain severe mental health conditions may require a more intensive and comprehensive treatment approach, such as medication or a combination of therapies.

Secondly, the success of CBT relies heavily on the therapeutic relationship and the client's willingness to actively participate in the process. Building a strong rapport and trust with the therapist is crucial for successful outcomes. Without a collaborative and trusting relationship, the effectiveness of CBT may be compromised.

Another limitation is that CBT primarily focuses on addressing the cognitive and behavioral aspects of mental health disorders. While this approach is effective for many individuals, it may not fully address underlying biological or physiological factors contributing to mental health issues. In such cases, a more comprehensive treatment plan that incorporates other modalities or interventions may be necessary.

It is also worth noting that CBT requires individuals to actively practice and apply the learned skills outside of therapy sessions. This can be challenging for some, especially if they face significant barriers or lack support in their daily lives. Without consistent practice and application of skills, the benefits of CBT may be limited.

Lastly, CBT is a structured and time-limited approach. While this structure can be beneficial for some individuals, it may not allow for the exploration of deeper underlying issues or ongoing support and maintenance of mental well-being. In cases where individuals require a more extended therapeutic intervention, other approaches or longer-term therapy may be more appropriate.

Despite these limitations, CBT remains a highly effective and evidence-based treatment for mental health conditions. By considering the individual's unique needs, preferences, and circumstances, mental health professionals can ensure the appropriate application of CBT and optimize treatment outcomes.

In conclusion, Cognitive Behavioral Therapy (CBT) is a powerful tool in the treatment of mental health disorders. Its effectiveness lies in its collaborative nature, empowering individuals to take an active role in their treatment and providing them with valuable coping skills. However, it is essential to recognize the limitations of CBT, such as its potential unsuitability for certain individuals, reliance on the therapeutic relationship, and its focus on cognitive and behavioral aspects. By acknowledging these limitations and adapting treatment plans accordingly, mental health professionals can maximize the potential of CBT and offer a comprehensive approach to client care.

Mindfulness-Based Interventions

Introduction to Mindfulness-Based Interventions

Mindfulness-Based Interventions (MBIs) have emerged as powerful approaches to improving mental health and well-being. These interventions draw from ancient contemplative practices and are designed to cultivate present-moment awareness, acceptance, and nonjudgmental attention. Mindfulness-based techniques have gained significant attention in recent years and have been widely adopted in various therapeutic settings.

The practice of mindfulness involves intentionally paying attention to thoughts, feelings, bodily sensations, and the surrounding environment, without judgment. It encourages individuals to observe their experiences as they arise, allowing them to develop a sense of self-awareness and promote a compassionate attitude towards themselves and others.

Understanding Mindfulness

Mindfulness is rooted in the teachings of ancient meditation practices, particularly in Buddhist traditions. It has been practiced for thousands of years as a way to cultivate inner peace, wisdom, and self-transformation. However, it was not until the late 20th century that mindfulness gained recognition in Western psychology and healthcare.

Jon Kabat-Zinn, a pioneer in the field, integrated mindfulness practices with cognitive-behavioral principles to develop Mindfulness-Based Stress Reduction (MBSR). MBSR was initially designed to support patients with chronic pain and later expanded to address a wide range of physical and mental health conditions. This program marked a significant milestone in the integration of mindfulness practices into mainstream healthcare.

Applications of Mindfulness-Based Interventions

Mindfulness-based interventions have shown promise in the treatment of various mental health disorders and promoting overall well-being. Some of the most well-known applications include:

1. **Stress reduction:** Mindfulness techniques help individuals manage stress by fostering the ability to observe their reactions and responses without becoming overwhelmed. This promotes adaptive coping strategies and reduces the harmful effects of chronic stress.

2. **Anxiety and depression:** MBIs have been found to be effective in reducing symptoms of anxiety and depression. By cultivating present-moment awareness, individuals learn to identify and challenge negative thinking patterns, regulate emotions, and increase self-compassion.

3. **Addiction and substance abuse:** Mindfulness helps individuals develop greater awareness of their cravings and habitual behaviors, improving their ability to make conscious choices. It also enhances emotional regulation and reduces the risk of relapse.

4. **Chronic pain management:** Mindfulness-based approaches have shown significant benefits for individuals with chronic pain, improving pain acceptance, and reducing emotional distress related to pain. It allows individuals to release resistance to their pain and cultivate a sense of resilience.

5. **Enhancing well-being:** Mindfulness practices cultivate a sense of gratitude, positive emotions, and overall well-being. They promote self-care, self-compassion, and strengthen resilience in the face of life challenges.

Benefits and Challenges of Mindfulness-Based Interventions

Mindfulness-based interventions offer numerous benefits for individuals seeking to improve their mental health and well-being. Some of the key advantages include:

- Improved emotional regulation: By cultivating present-moment awareness, individuals develop the ability to observe their thoughts and emotions without judgment. This allows for a more skillful response to difficult emotions and reduces emotional reactivity.

- Stress reduction: Mindfulness helps individuals manage stress by increasing awareness of stress triggers and providing effective coping strategies. Regular practice can lead to improved resilience and a greater sense of calm and well-being.

- Increased self-compassion: Mindfulness encourages individuals to develop a compassionate attitude towards themselves and others. This fosters self-acceptance, self-care, and nurtures more positive relationships.

- Improved cognitive functioning: Research suggests that mindfulness training can enhance attention, memory, and cognitive flexibility. Individuals may experience improved problem-solving skills, creativity, and overall cognitive performance.

However, like any therapeutic intervention, mindfulness-based practices also come with some challenges:

- Commitment and consistency: Mindfulness requires regular practice to yield significant benefits. Developing a consistent practice can be challenging, especially in today's fast-paced and demanding world.

- Initial discomfort: Some individuals may initially find it challenging to be present with their thoughts and emotions. It may bring up uncomfortable sensations or resistance. However, with time and practice, most individuals find it easier to navigate these experiences.

- Skillful guidance: Mindfulness practices are best learned under the guidance of a qualified instructor who can address individual needs and provide appropriate support. Finding a skilled teacher or therapist can be crucial in maximizing the benefits of mindfulness-based interventions.

In conclusion, mindfulness-based interventions are valuable tools for improving mental health and overall well-being. By integrating ancient contemplative practices with modern psychology, these interventions provide individuals with practical skills to navigate the challenges of everyday life, enhancing resilience, self-compassion, and emotional regulation. With commitment and practice, mindfulness can be a transformative force in promoting mental health and well-being.

Applications of Mindfulness-Based Interventions in Mental Health

Mindfulness-based interventions (MBIs) have gained significant recognition in the field of mental health due to their effectiveness in promoting overall wellbeing. These interventions involve incorporating mindfulness practices, such as meditation and body awareness, into therapeutic approaches. MBIs have been found to be beneficial for a wide range of mental health conditions, and their applications continue to expand. In this section, we will explore some of the key applications of mindfulness-based interventions in mental health.

Anxiety Disorders

Anxiety disorders, such as generalized anxiety disorder, panic disorder, and social anxiety disorder, can significantly impact a person's quality of life. MBIs have shown promise in reducing anxiety symptoms and improving overall functioning in individuals with these disorders. Mindfulness-based stress reduction (MBSR) and mindfulness-based cognitive therapy (MBCT) are two widely used interventions for anxiety.

MBSR involves training individuals to pay attention to the present moment, non-judgmentally, through mindfulness meditation and body awareness exercises. This helps individuals become more aware of their anxious thoughts and physical sensations, allowing them to respond to them in a non-reactive manner. MBCT combines mindfulness practices with elements of cognitive therapy to help individuals identify and challenge maladaptive thought patterns associated with anxiety.

Example: Sarah, a 32-year-old woman with social anxiety disorder, participates in an eight-week MBCT program. Through mindfulness practices, she becomes more aware of her self-critical thoughts and the physical sensations that arise in social situations. As she practices responding to these thoughts and sensations with acceptance and non-judgment, Sarah experiences a reduction in her anxiety symptoms and an increased ability to engage in social interactions.

Depression

Depression is a prevalent mental health condition characterized by persistent feelings of sadness, hopelessness, and a loss of interest in activities. Mindfulness-based interventions have been found to be effective in reducing depressive symptoms and preventing relapse in individuals with a history of depression.

Mindfulness-based cognitive therapy (MBCT) combines mindfulness practices with cognitive therapy techniques to help individuals recognize and disengage from negative thought patterns associated with depression. By practicing non-reactivity and acceptance of these thoughts and emotions, individuals can cultivate a sense of self-compassion and develop more adaptive coping strategies.

Example: John, a 45-year-old man who has experienced several episodes of depression, participates in an MBCT program. Through mindfulness practices, he becomes aware of the repetitive negative thoughts and self-critical beliefs that contribute to his depressive symptoms. With continued practice, John learns to observe these thoughts without judgment and develops the ability to respond to them in a more compassionate and constructive manner. As a result, he experiences a reduction in his depressive symptoms and gains a greater sense of control over his mood.

Stress Reduction

Stress is a common experience that can negatively impact mental health and overall well-being. Mindfulness-based interventions have been shown to be effective in reducing stress and promoting relaxation. MBSR, in particular, is often used as an intervention to manage stress-related conditions.

MBSR teaches individuals to cultivate moment-to-moment awareness of their thoughts, emotions, and bodily sensations. By becoming more present and accepting of their experiences, individuals can develop greater resilience to stress and enhance their ability to cope with challenging situations. MBSR often includes practices such as body scan meditation, mindful movement, and mindfulness of breath.

Example: Lisa, a 50-year-old woman experiencing high levels of work-related stress, enrolls in an MBSR course. As she learns to bring mindful awareness to her thoughts and physical sensations, Lisa becomes more attuned to the early signs of stress in her body. With regular practice, she develops a greater capacity to respond to stressors with calmness and clarity. As a result, Lisa experiences a reduction in her overall stress levels and an improved sense of well-being.

Substance Use Disorders

Mindfulness-based interventions have been successfully integrated into the treatment of substance use disorders, such as alcohol and drug addiction. These interventions help individuals develop greater awareness and acceptance of their cravings, emotions, and physical sensations associated with substance use.

Mindfulness-based relapse prevention (MBRP) is an evidence-based intervention that combines mindfulness practices with cognitive-behavioral strategies to prevent relapse. By cultivating non-judgmental awareness and using mindfulness techniques to navigate cravings and triggers, individuals develop the skills needed to effectively cope with the challenges of recovery.

Example: Mark, a 28-year-old man in recovery from alcohol addiction, participates in an MBRP program. Through mindfulness practices, he learns to observe his cravings without automatically acting on them. By developing an attitude of acceptance and curiosity towards his cravings, Mark becomes more skilled at understanding the underlying emotional and physical triggers that contribute to his substance use. As a result, he is better equipped to manage these triggers and maintain his sobriety.

Attention-Deficit Hyperactivity Disorder (ADHD)

ADHD is a neurodevelopmental disorder characterized by symptoms such as inattention, hyperactivity, and impulsivity. Mindfulness-based interventions have shown promise in improving the core symptoms of ADHD and enhancing self-regulation skills.

Mindfulness training for ADHD involves cultivating present-moment awareness and bringing attention to one's experiences without judgment. By practicing mindfulness, individuals with ADHD can enhance their ability to focus, regulate their impulses, and improve emotional self-regulation.

Example: Alex, a 10-year-old boy diagnosed with ADHD, participates in a mindfulness-based intervention tailored for children. Through mindfulness exercises and guided meditations, Alex learns to bring intentional focus to his thoughts, emotions, and actions. As he practices mindfulness, Alex experiences improved attention and impulse control, leading to better academic performance and an increased sense of self-efficacy.

Caveats and Considerations

While mindfulness-based interventions can be highly beneficial, it is essential to consider individual differences and potential challenges when implementing these approaches. Some individuals may find it difficult to sit still for mindfulness practices or may struggle with initial discomfort when facing their thoughts and emotions. Creating a safe and supportive environment, providing guidance and adaptations as needed, can help overcome these challenges.

Additionally, it is important to note that while mindfulness-based interventions can be effective on their own, they are often most beneficial when integrated with other evidence-based treatments. Collaborating with mental health professionals and tailoring interventions to the specific needs of individuals ensures comprehensive and effective care.

Resources

- *The Mindful Way Workbook: An 8-Week Program to Free Yourself from Depression and Emotional Distress* by John D. Teasdale, J. Mark G. Williams, and Zindel V. Segal - *Full Catastrophe Living: Using the Wisdom of Your Body and Mind to Face Stress, Pain, and Illness* by Jon Kabat-Zinn - *The Dialectical Behavior Therapy Skills Workbook: Practical DBT Exercises for Learning Mindfulness, Interpersonal Effectiveness, Emotion Regulation & Distress Tolerance* by Matthew McKay, Jeffrey C. Wood, and Jeffrey Brantley - *The Science of Meditation: How to Change Your Brain, Mind and Body* by Daniel Goleman and Richard J. Davidson

Conclusion

Mindfulness-based interventions have emerged as valuable tools in promoting mental health and wellbeing. Their applications in various mental health conditions are supported by a growing body of research. By incorporating mindfulness practices into therapeutic approaches, individuals can develop greater awareness, self-compassion, and resilience, leading to improved mental health outcomes. Continued research, collaboration, and the integration of MBIs into clinical practice will shape the future of mental health care.

Benefits and Challenges of Mindfulness-Based Interventions

Mindfulness-based interventions (MBIs) have gained considerable recognition and popularity in recent years for their potential to promote mental health and overall well-being. These interventions draw from the principles of mindfulness, which involve paying attention to the present moment with an attitude of non-judgmental awareness. In this section, we will explore the benefits and challenges of MBIs, highlighting their potential impact on mental health.

Benefits of Mindfulness-Based Interventions

1. **Stress reduction:** One of the primary benefits of MBIs is their ability to reduce stress levels. Research has shown that practicing mindfulness can help individuals

develop a greater capacity to manage stress and respond effectively to challenging situations. By cultivating a non-reactive and compassionate attitude towards one's experiences, mindfulness helps individuals break free from the cycle of stress and develop a sense of inner calm and resilience.

2. **Emotional regulation**: Mindfulness practice involves observing and acknowledging emotions without judgment. This allows individuals to develop greater emotional awareness and regulation. Through MBIs, individuals learn to identify and accept their emotions, reducing emotional reactivity and promoting adaptive coping strategies. This can be particularly beneficial for individuals struggling with mood disorders, anxiety, or emotional dysregulation.

3. **Improved cognitive functioning**: Regular practice of mindfulness has been associated with improved cognitive functions such as attention, working memory, and executive functioning. By training individuals to redirect their attention to the present moment, mindfulness helps reduce cognitive distractions and enhance focus. This can be valuable for individuals experiencing difficulties with concentration or cognitive decline.

4. **Enhanced self-awareness and self-compassion**: Mindfulness cultivates self-awareness, allowing individuals to develop a clearer understanding of their thoughts, feelings, and bodily sensations. This heightened self-awareness promotes self-compassion, as individuals learn to accept themselves without judgment. By cultivating self-compassion, MBIs foster a kinder and more supportive relationship with oneself, leading to improved self-esteem and overall well-being.

5. **Improved interpersonal relationships**: Mindfulness practice encourages individuals to be fully present and attentive in their interactions with others. This fosters better communication, empathy, and understanding in relationships. By engaging in active listening and practicing non-reactivity, individuals can navigate conflicts more effectively and promote healthier, more meaningful connections with others.

Challenges of Mindfulness-Based Interventions

While MBIs offer numerous benefits, it is important to acknowledge and address the challenges that individuals may encounter during their mindfulness practice. Awareness of these challenges helps individuals make informed decisions about their participation in such interventions and can support their engagement in a meaningful way.

1. **Difficulties with sustained practice**: Consistency and commitment to regular mindfulness practice can be challenging for individuals with busy schedules or competing priorities. Developing a sustained practice requires discipline and

motivation. Educating individuals about the importance of regular practice, providing support in developing a routine, and offering flexible options for practice can help address this challenge.

2. **Initial discomfort with being present:** In the early stages of mindfulness practice, individuals may experience discomfort or restlessness when faced with sitting quietly and focusing on the present moment. This discomfort is natural, as the mind tends to wander and resist the practice. Educating participants about the normalcy of these experiences and providing guidance on working through initial discomfort can help individuals persist in their practice.

3. **Cultural and religious concerns:** Mindfulness-based interventions have roots in Buddhist traditions, which may raise cultural or religious concerns for some individuals. It is important to offer MBIs in a secular and inclusive manner, making them accessible and relevant to individuals from diverse cultural and religious backgrounds. Highlighting the evidence-based nature of MBIs and focusing on the universal principles of mindfulness can help alleviate these concerns.

4. **Challenges in applying mindfulness in daily life:** While individuals may find it relatively easy to practice mindfulness in a controlled environment, transferring mindfulness skills to daily life can be challenging. Applying mindfulness in real-life situations requires effort and a shift in mindset. Integrating mindfulness into daily routines and providing guidance on applying mindfulness techniques in various contexts can support individuals in translating their practice into everyday life.

5. **Discomfort with difficult emotions:** Mindfulness practice involves cultivating an accepting and non-judgmental stance towards all experiences, including difficult emotions. This can be challenging for individuals who are not accustomed to acknowledging or accepting their negative emotions. Encouraging self-compassion, providing psychoeducation on emotions, and teaching specific mindfulness techniques to manage difficult emotions can support individuals in their mindfulness journey.

By addressing these challenges and capitalizing on the numerous benefits, mindfulness-based interventions can be a powerful tool for promoting mental health and well-being. It is important to customize interventions to individual needs, provide ongoing support, and promote a non-judgmental and inclusive environment for individuals to fully engage in their mindfulness practice.

Art Therapy

Overview of Art Therapy

Art therapy is a creative and expressive therapeutic modality that utilizes various art mediums to support the healing process and promote psychological well-being. It involves the use of visual arts, such as drawing, painting, sculpture, and collage, as well as other art forms like music, dance, and poetry. The aim of art therapy is to enable individuals to explore their emotions, thoughts, and experiences in a non-verbal and symbolic manner.

Theoretical Foundations

Art therapy is grounded in several theoretical frameworks, including psychodynamic, humanistic, and cognitive-behavioral theories. Psychodynamic theory, influenced by the work of Sigmund Freud, emphasizes the role of the unconscious mind and the exploration of inner conflicts through the art-making process. Humanistic theories, such as person-centered and gestalt approaches, highlight the importance of self-expression, personal growth, and self-actualization. Cognitive-behavioral theories focus on the relationship between thoughts, feelings, and behaviors, and how art-making can help individuals challenge and reframe their cognitive patterns.

Key Principles

Art therapy is guided by several key principles that inform its practice:

1. **Creative process:** The emphasis is on the process of creation rather than the product. The art therapist encourages the individual to freely express themselves without judgment or evaluation.

2. **Symbolism and metaphor:** Artistic expression can tap into the unconscious and reveal hidden emotions and thoughts through symbolic representation. Artwork is often interpreted metaphorically to gain insight into the individual's internal world.

3. **Non-verbal communication:** Art provides a means for communication that goes beyond words. It allows individuals to express complex feelings and experiences that may be difficult to articulate verbally.

4. **Empowerment and self-discovery:** Art therapy aims to empower individuals by providing a safe and non-threatening space for self-exploration. Through creativity, individuals can gain a deeper understanding of themselves and develop a sense of agency.

5. **Integration and insight:** The art-making process helps integrate cognitive, emotional, and sensory experiences, enabling individuals to gain insight into their thoughts, feelings, and behaviors. This integration promotes personal growth and enhances self-awareness.

Applications of Art Therapy

Art therapy is used across a wide range of populations and settings, including clinical, educational, and community-based contexts. It is effective in addressing various mental health concerns, such as:

- **Trauma and PTSD:** Art therapy can help individuals process traumatic experiences, reduce distressing symptoms, and foster post-traumatic growth. The use of art-making provides a safe and structured approach to explore and integrate traumatic memories.

- **Anxiety and depression:** Art therapy offers a creative outlet for individuals to express and manage their emotions. The process of art-making can be soothing and provide a sense of control, reducing anxiety and improving mood.

- **Self-esteem and body image issues:** Art therapy supports individuals in developing a positive self-image and improving self-esteem. Through art, individuals can explore and challenge negative self-perceptions, promoting self-acceptance and self-love.

- **Relationship and interpersonal difficulties:** Art therapy can facilitate communication and expression of emotions within relationships. It can help individuals explore past and current relational patterns, promote empathy, and enhance social skills.

- **Stress management:** Engaging in art-making can be a grounding and calming practice that reduces stress and promotes relaxation. It provides a means for self-care and self-expression, allowing individuals to explore and process their stressors.

Overall, art therapy offers a unique and powerful approach to healing and self-discovery by harnessing the creative process. Its interdisciplinary nature allows for integration with other therapeutic modalities and enhances the overall well-being of individuals. Art therapists are trained professionals who combine their knowledge of psychology, creativity, and the therapeutic process to guide individuals on their journey towards self-growth and transformation.

Resources and Professional Organizations

For those interested in learning more about art therapy or pursuing a career in the field, there are several resources and professional organizations available:

- **American Art Therapy Association (AATA):** The AATA is a leading professional organization that provides resources, education, and advocacy for art therapists. Their website offers information on training programs, professional development opportunities, and research in the field.
- **International Expressive Arts Therapy Association (IEATA):** IEATA is a global organization that promotes the use of expressive arts in therapy and education. Their website provides access to publications, conferences, and training opportunities for individuals interested in expressive arts therapy.
- **Books and Journals:** There are numerous books and journals dedicated to art therapy theory, practice, and research. Some recommended texts include "Art Therapy: Theories and Techniques" by Judith A. Rubin and "The Handbook of Art Therapy" edited by Cathy A. Malchiodi.
- **Art Materials and Supplies:** Various art supply stores offer a wide range of materials suitable for art therapy. These include paints, brushes, clay, and other art-making tools. It is important to ensure the safety and appropriateness of materials for therapeutic use.

Art therapy is a dynamic and evolving field that continues to contribute to the mental health and well-being of diverse individuals and communities. By harnessing the power of creativity and self-expression, art therapy offers a transformative approach to support healing, personal growth, and positive change.

The Therapeutic Role of Art in Mental Health

Art has long been recognized for its ability to evoke emotions, express thoughts, and capture the human experience. In recent years, the therapeutic benefits of engaging in art-making activities have gained significant attention in the field of mental health. This section explores the therapeutic role of art in promoting mental health and wellbeing, and discusses its applications, effectiveness, and underlying mechanisms.

Art Therapy: An Overview

Art therapy is a specialized, evidence-based form of therapy that integrates the creative process of art-making with psychological counseling. It is facilitated by trained art therapists who provide a safe and supportive space for individuals to explore and express themselves through various art media, such as painting, drawing, sculpture, and collage. The unique combination of art and therapy enables individuals to tap into their inner resources, enhance self-awareness, and foster personal growth.

The use of art as a therapeutic tool dates back to ancient times, where it was employed as a means of self-expression and healing. However, art therapy as a distinct discipline emerged in the mid-20th century with the pioneering work of artists and mental health professionals. Today, art therapy is recognized as an effective intervention for individuals of all ages and backgrounds, including those with mental health disorders, trauma, or other emotional challenges.

Applications of Art Therapy in Mental Health

Art therapy can be applied in a variety of mental health settings, including hospitals, clinics, schools, and community centers. It is utilized as a standalone treatment modality or as an adjunct to traditional talk therapy. Art therapists work collaboratively with their clients to identify and address specific therapeutic goals, which may include:

- Enhancing self-expression and communication: Art provides an alternative means of expression for individuals who may struggle to verbally articulate their emotions or experiences. Through art-making, clients can communicate their thoughts and feelings that might otherwise remain unexpressed.

- Promoting emotional healing and self-discovery: Engaging in the creative process can facilitate emotional release and catharsis. Art therapy allows individuals to explore their inner world, gain insights into their emotions, and develop a deeper understanding of themselves.

- Managing stress and anxiety: The act of creating art stimulates the relaxation response, helping to reduce stress and anxiety. The repetitive nature of certain art techniques, such as coloring or collage, can induce a meditative state, promoting a sense of calm and mental clarity.

- Building self-esteem and confidence: Art-making provides opportunities for success and accomplishment, fostering a sense of pride and self-worth. The experience of creating something meaningful and aesthetically pleasing can boost self-esteem and confidence.

- Resolving trauma and processing grief: Art therapy can assist individuals in healing from traumatic experiences and navigating the complex emotions associated with grief and loss. The symbolic nature of art allows for the exploration of traumatic memories and the facilitation of the healing process.

Effectiveness and Limitations of Art Therapy

Numerous research studies have demonstrated the effectiveness of art therapy in improving mental health outcomes. For example, a meta-analysis conducted by Stuckey and Nobel (2010) found that art therapy significantly reduced symptoms of anxiety, depression, and trauma-related distress across various populations. Additionally, art therapy has been shown to enhance coping skills, increase self-awareness, and foster personal growth.

It is important to note that art therapy is not a panacea and may not be suitable for everyone. Some individuals may feel uncomfortable with the creative process or find it challenging to express themselves through art. Flexibility and individualization are key components of art therapy, allowing for adaptations and modifications to meet the unique needs of each client.

The Mechanisms Behind Art Therapy

The therapeutic benefits of art therapy can be attributed to several underlying mechanisms. Firstly, the act of engaging in art-making activates the brain's reward system, releasing neurotransmitters such as dopamine and endorphins that contribute to feelings of pleasure and well-being. This neurochemical response can enhance mood and alleviate symptoms of depression and anxiety.

Secondly, art therapy promotes mindfulness and present-moment awareness. When individuals immerse themselves in the creative process, they enter a state of flow, characterized by deep concentration and a loss of self-consciousness. This meditative state helps individuals engage fully in the present moment, fostering relaxation and stress reduction.

Additionally, art-making can serve as a form of non-verbal communication, allowing individuals to bypass cognitive defenses and access deeper emotional experiences. The symbolic nature of art provides a safe distance for individuals to explore and externalize difficult emotions, memories, and conflicts. Through the metaphorical language of art, clients can gain new insights and perspectives, leading to greater self-understanding and personal growth.

Examples and Resources

Art therapy encompasses a wide range of techniques and approaches that can be tailored to the specific needs and preferences of individuals. Some examples of art therapy interventions include:

- Creating a visual journal: Encouraging individuals to keep a visual diary where they can freely express their thoughts, feelings, and experiences through art and writing.

- Painting emotions: Using colors, shapes, and textures to represent different emotions and exploring their meanings and associations.

- Group collage: Engaging in collaborative collage-making activities to promote social connection, communication, and shared experiences.

- Sculpting with clay: Providing a tactile and sensory experience for individuals to express and externalize their emotions or create symbolic representations of themselves.

Art therapy resources are widely available, including books, online courses, and professional organizations. The American Art Therapy Association (AATA) and the International Expressive Arts Therapy Association (IEATA) are valuable sources of information, research, and guidelines for both practitioners and individuals interested in exploring art therapy.

Caveats and Considerations

While art therapy has shown promising results, it is essential to recognize its limitations and consider certain caveats. Importantly, art therapy should not be viewed as a replacement for conventional mental health treatment, but rather as a complementary approach that can be integrated into a comprehensive treatment plan.

Art therapists must adhere to ethical guidelines and possess appropriate qualifications and training. The expertise and skill of the therapist in facilitating the creative process, interpreting the artwork, and creating a safe and supportive therapeutic environment are crucial factors impacting the effectiveness of art therapy.

Moreover, cultural considerations must be taken into account to ensure inclusivity and sensitivity in the practice of art therapy. Different cultures may have varying beliefs and attitudes towards art and its use in therapy. Art therapists need to embrace cultural diversity and adapt their approaches accordingly to respect and honor clients' cultural backgrounds.

Exercise: Exploring Art as a Therapeutic Tool

Take a few moments to reflect on the following exercise:

1. Find a quiet and comfortable space where you can engage in a creative activity.
2. Gather art materials of your choice, such as paper, markers, paints, or clay.
3. Set a specific intention or therapeutic goal for this exercise. It could be expressing an emotion, exploring a personal challenge, or simply connecting with your inner self.
4. Engage in the art-making process, allowing yourself to freely express and explore your thoughts and feelings. Let go of any expectations or judgments and focus on the process rather than the end product.
5. Take a moment to reflect on your artwork. What thoughts, emotions, or insights arise? How did engaging in this creative activity make you feel?

Remember, this exercise is for personal exploration and self-reflection. There are no right or wrong answers, and your artwork is a reflection of your unique experience.

Conclusion

Art therapy offers a unique and impactful approach to promoting mental health and wellbeing. By harnessing the power of creativity, individuals can tap into their inner resources, express themselves authentically, and find healing and personal growth. The therapeutic role of art in mental health is increasingly recognized and valued, providing individuals with unique opportunities for self-exploration, emotional healing, and empowerment.

Applications and Effectiveness of Art Therapy

Art therapy is a form of expressive therapy that utilizes various art forms, such as painting, drawing, sculpture, and collage, as a means of communication and self-expression. It is a therapeutic approach that can be used with individuals of all ages and backgrounds, and it has been found to be effective in addressing a wide range of mental health concerns. In this section, we will explore the applications and effectiveness of art therapy in different contexts.

Applications of Art Therapy

Art therapy can be applied in various settings, including clinical settings, schools, community centers, and rehabilitation facilities. It can be used as a standalone therapy or in combination with other therapeutic modalities, depending on the needs and goals of the individual. Some common applications of art therapy include:

1. **Individual therapy**: Art therapy can be used as a form of individual therapy to help individuals explore and process their emotions, thoughts, and experiences. Through art-making, individuals can express and communicate their innermost feelings that may be difficult to put into words.

2. **Group therapy**: Art therapy can also be conducted in a group setting, where individuals have the opportunity to share their artwork and engage in discussions. Group art therapy provides a supportive and collaborative environment, allowing participants to connect with others who may be experiencing similar challenges.

3. **Trauma treatment**: Art therapy has been widely used in trauma treatment, as it provides a nonverbal medium for individuals to express and process their traumatic experiences. Art-making can help individuals reconnect with their emotions, regain a sense of control, and promote healing and growth.

4. **Children and adolescents**: Art therapy is particularly effective with children and adolescents, as it allows them to express themselves freely and creatively. It can help children and adolescents explore their identities, build self-esteem, develop coping skills, and address various behavioral and emotional challenges.

5. **Geriatric population**: Art therapy has shown positive outcomes in working with the elderly population, particularly those with dementia and Alzheimer's disease. Engaging in art-making can stimulate cognitive functioning, enhance memory recall, and improve overall well-being and quality of life.

Effectiveness of Art Therapy

Research has consistently shown the effectiveness of art therapy in various mental health domains. Some key findings include:

1. **Reducing symptoms of anxiety and depression:** Art therapy has been found to reduce symptoms of anxiety and depression in individuals of all ages. The creative process involved in art-making can serve as a form of self-soothing and stress relief, promoting relaxation and emotional well-being.

2. **Enhancing self-expression and self-awareness:** Art therapy provides a safe and supportive space for individuals to express themselves authentically and explore their inner worlds. Through art-making, individuals can gain insight into their emotions, thoughts, and behaviors, fostering self-awareness and personal growth.

3. **Improving emotional regulation:** Engaging in art therapy can help individuals regulate their emotions by providing a medium to externalize and process difficult feelings. It allows for the exploration of emotional experiences in a non-threatening and non-judgmental manner.

4. **Promoting insight and problem-solving:** Art therapy can facilitate problem-solving skills by encouraging individuals to explore new perspectives and alternative solutions through their artwork. The creative process can stimulate imagination and encourage flexible thinking, leading to increased problem-solving abilities.

5. **Enhancing overall well-being:** Regular engagement in art therapy has been associated with increased overall well-being and quality of life. It has been shown to reduce stress, increase self-esteem, promote relaxation, and cultivate a sense of purpose and meaning.

Despite the growing evidence supporting its effectiveness, it is important to note that art therapy is not a substitute for traditional therapy approaches or medication when necessary. It is typically used as a complementary therapy to support and enhance other therapeutic interventions.

Case Example

To illustrate the applications and effectiveness of art therapy, consider the following case example:

Sarah, a 35-year-old woman, has been struggling with symptoms of anxiety and low self-esteem. She finds it challenging to articulate her emotions verbally and often feels overwhelmed. Her therapist incorporates art therapy into her treatment plan to provide an alternative means of expression.

Through art therapy sessions, Sarah engages in various art activities, such as creating collages and painting. She discovers that the creative process allows her to access and express her emotions in a nonverbal way. Sarah starts to explore themes of fear, self-doubt, and resilience in her artwork, and through discussions with her therapist, she gains new insights into her thoughts and feelings.

Over time, Sarah's anxiety symptoms lessen, and she develops a greater sense of self-awareness and self-acceptance. Art therapy becomes a vital tool in her ongoing mental health journey, allowing her to continue exploring and processing her experiences beyond the therapy sessions.

Resources for Art Therapy

If you are interested in learning more about art therapy or incorporating art-based techniques into your practice, the following resources can be helpful:

1. *Art Therapy Sourcebook* by Cathy Malchiodi provides an overview of art therapy principles, techniques, and applications.
2. The *American Art Therapy Association* (www.arttherapy.org) offers information on training programs, research, and resources for professionals and individuals seeking art therapy services.
3. The *International Expressive Arts Therapy Association* (www.ieata.org) provides resources, training programs, and a global network for professionals practicing various forms of expressive arts therapy.
4. Local art therapy workshops and conferences offer opportunities to learn from experienced art therapists and connect with others in the field.

Remember, incorporating art therapy into your practice requires appropriate training and understanding of ethical guidelines. Collaboration with certified art therapists or seeking specialized training can ensure the safe and effective integration of art therapy techniques into your work.

In conclusion, art therapy is a powerful and versatile therapeutic approach that offers a range of applications and proven effectiveness. By engaging in the creative process, individuals can tap into their inner resources, improve emotional well-being, and foster personal growth.

Yoga and Meditation

Introduction to Yoga and Meditation

Yoga and meditation are ancient practices that have been used for centuries to promote physical, mental, and spiritual well-being. In recent years, these practices have gained widespread recognition and have become an integral part of many people's lives. In this section, we will explore the fundamentals of yoga and meditation, their benefits, and how they can be incorporated into a modern lifestyle.

The Philosophy of Yoga

Yoga originated in ancient India and is rooted in the philosophy of Hinduism and Buddhism. It combines physical postures, breathing exercises, and meditation techniques to unite the body, mind, and spirit. The word "yoga" is derived from the Sanskrit word "yuj," which means to join or unite.

At its core, yoga aims to create harmony between the physical and mental aspects of an individual. It emphasizes the importance of self-awareness, self-discipline, and self-realization. The practice of yoga is not limited to physical exercise; it encompasses a holistic approach to life, encompassing ethical principles, moral values, and a conscious way of living.

Benefits of Yoga

The practice of yoga offers numerous physical, mental, and emotional benefits. Some of the key benefits include:

1. Physical well-being: Yoga improves flexibility, strength, and balance. It helps to tone the muscles, improve posture, and increase overall body awareness. Regular yoga practice can also alleviate chronic pain, reduce inflammation, and enhance cardiovascular health.

2. Stress reduction: One of the primary benefits of yoga is its ability to reduce stress and promote relaxation. The combination of breathing exercises, physical movement, and mindfulness helps to calm the nervous system, lower cortisol levels, and induce a state of tranquility and inner peace.

3. Mental clarity and focus: Regular yoga practice enhances mental clarity, improves concentration, and increases focus. The practice of meditation, which is an integral part of yoga, helps to quiet the mind, reduce mental chatter, and enhance emotional well-being.

4. Emotional balance: Yoga cultivates emotional awareness and helps to regulate emotions. It provides a safe space for introspection and self-reflection, allowing individuals to develop a deeper understanding of their thoughts, feelings, and behaviors. This self-awareness can lead to a greater sense of emotional balance and harmony.

Different Styles of Yoga

There are several different styles of yoga, each with its own unique emphasis and approach. Some of the most popular styles include:

1. Hatha Yoga: Hatha yoga is a gentle and slow-paced form of yoga that focuses on physical postures (asanas) and breathing techniques (pranayama). It is suitable for all fitness levels and is often used as a starting point for beginners.

2. Vinyasa Yoga: Vinyasa yoga is characterized by flowing movements and transitions between poses, synchronized with breath. It is a dynamic and energetic style of yoga that helps to build strength, flexibility, and endurance.

3. Ashtanga Yoga: Ashtanga yoga is a rigorous and structured style of yoga that follows a specific sequence of postures. It involves synchronized breathing and continuous movement, making it a physically demanding practice.

4. Bikram Yoga: Bikram yoga, also known as hot yoga, is practiced in a heated room. It consists of a series of 26 postures and two breathing exercises. The heat helps to loosen the muscles, promote detoxification, and increase flexibility.

5. Kundalini Yoga: Kundalini yoga focuses on awakening the dormant spiritual energy (kundalini) within the body. It combines physical postures, breathing exercises, chanting, and meditation to stimulate spiritual growth and self-awareness.

Incorporating Meditation

Meditation is an essential component of yoga practice and can be practiced independently as well. It involves focusing the mind and cultivating a state of deep relaxation and heightened awareness. Meditation techniques vary, but they generally involve finding a comfortable seated position, focusing on the breath or a specific object, and observing the thoughts and sensations that arise without judgment.

Regular meditation practice has been linked to many benefits, including stress reduction, improved concentration, emotional well-being, and increased self-awareness. It can be practiced by anyone, regardless of age or physical fitness level, and can easily be incorporated into a daily routine.

Resources and Tips

If you are interested in exploring yoga and meditation further, here are some resources and tips to get you started:

1. Find a qualified instructor: It is advisable to learn yoga and meditation from a qualified instructor who can guide you through the practices and ensure correct alignment and technique.

2. Start with beginner-friendly classes: If you are new to yoga, start with beginner-friendly classes that focus on the basics and gradually progress to more advanced levels as you become more comfortable.

3. Create a dedicated space: Set aside a quiet and peaceful space in your home where you can practice yoga and meditation without distractions. Decorate it with items that inspire and relax you, such as candles, incense, or plants.

4. Establish a regular practice: Consistency is key when it comes to yoga and meditation. Set aside a specific time each day for your practice, even if it's just a few minutes in the beginning.

5. Explore different styles: Don't be afraid to explore different styles of yoga and meditation to find what resonates with you. There is no one-size-fits-all approach, and it's important to find practices that align with your needs and preferences.

Remember, yoga and meditation are not competitive sports. Listen to your body, respect your limits, and focus on your own journey. With regular practice and an open mind, you can experience the transformative power of yoga and meditation in your life.

Conclusion

Yoga and meditation offer a holistic approach to mental health and well-being. By incorporating these practices into your daily life, you can improve physical fitness, reduce stress, increase self-awareness, and cultivate inner peace. Whether you are a beginner or an experienced practitioner, the benefits of yoga and meditation are available to everyone. Embrace the journey, explore different styles, and discover the transformative power of these ancient practices.

The Mind-Body Connection in Mental Health

The mind-body connection plays a vital role in mental health and well-being. It refers to the intricate relationship between our thoughts, emotions, and physical body. Understanding this connection is crucial for developing effective interventions and treatments for mental health disorders. In this section, we will explore the various aspects of the mind-body connection and its significance in promoting mental wellness.

Background

The concept of the mind-body connection has been recognized for centuries, with ancient healing traditions such as Ayurveda and Traditional Chinese Medicine emphasizing the interconnection between the mind and the body. However, it is only in recent years that scientific research has provided compelling evidence for this connection.

Principles of the Mind-Body Connection

At the core of the mind-body connection is the understanding that our thoughts, emotions, and physical sensations are deeply intertwined. Several key principles underline this connection:

1. **Psychosomatic Influence:** Our mental and emotional states can have a profound impact on our physical well-being. For example, stress and anxiety can manifest as physical symptoms like muscle tension, headaches, or digestive issues.

2. **Biological Pathways:** The mind-body connection operates through various biological pathways, including the nervous system, the endocrine system, and the immune system. These systems constantly communicate and influence one another, impacting our overall health.

3. **Emotional Regulation:** Emotions play a crucial role in the mind-body connection. Our ability to recognize, express, and regulate our emotions influences our mental and physical well-being. When emotional regulation is compromised, it can lead to negative health outcomes.

4. **Neuroplasticity:** The brain has the remarkable ability to change and adapt throughout our lives. Neuroplasticity is the phenomenon by which the brain's structure and function can be modified in response to our experiences, thoughts, and emotions. This process highlights the dynamic nature of the mind-body connection.

Impact of the Mind-Body Connection on Mental Health

The mind-body connection has a significant impact on mental health. Here are some key ways in which it influences mental well-being:

- **Stress and Anxiety:** Chronic stress and anxiety can result in physical symptoms such as elevated heart rate, muscle tension, and weakened immune function. Additionally, they can contribute to the development and exacerbation of mental health disorders like depression and anxiety disorders.

- **Psychosomatic Disorders:** Psychological distress can manifest as physical symptoms and disorders. Conditions like irritable bowel syndrome, tension headaches, and fibromyalgia are examples of psychosomatic disorders where the mind-body connection is evident.

- **Emotional Regulation:** Difficulties in regulating emotions can lead to mental health challenges. Individuals who struggle with emotional regulation may experience heightened stress levels, mood disturbances, and a decreased ability to cope with life's challenges.

- **Resilience and Well-being:** Cultivating a positive mind-body connection can contribute to resilience and overall well-being. A strong mind-body connection supports emotional balance, enhances coping skills, and fosters a sense of purpose and meaning in life.

Interventions Targeting the Mind-Body Connection

Recognizing the power of the mind-body connection, various interventions have been developed to promote mental health and well-being. Here are some examples:

- **Mindfulness-Based Practices:** Mindfulness-based interventions, such as mindfulness meditation and yoga, emphasize cultivating present-moment awareness. These practices help individuals develop a deeper connection between their thoughts, emotions, and bodily sensations, leading to greater self-awareness and stress reduction.

- **Physical Activity and Exercise:** Engaging in regular physical activity and exercise supports the mind-body connection by releasing endorphins, reducing stress hormones, and promoting neural plasticity. Exercise has been shown to alleviate symptoms of depression and anxiety, enhance mood, and improve overall mental well-being.

- **Cognitive-Behavioral Therapy (CBT):** CBT is a widely used therapeutic approach that recognizes the interplay between thoughts, emotions, and behaviors. By identifying and modifying negative thought patterns, CBT aims to promote positive emotional experiences and improve mental health outcomes.

- **Expressive Arts Therapies:** Art-based interventions, such as art therapy and music therapy, provide avenues for self-expression and emotional exploration. These therapeutic modalities leverage creative processes to enhance self-awareness, emotional regulation, and overall psychological well-being.

Case Study: Mindfulness-Based Stress Reduction

To further illustrate the practical application of the mind-body connection, let's consider the case of Sarah, a 35-year-old woman experiencing chronic stress and anxiety. Sarah decides to enroll in a mindfulness-based stress reduction (MBSR) program.

Throughout the program, Sarah learns mindfulness meditation techniques, body scans, and gentle yoga exercises. By practicing these techniques, she becomes more aware of the connection between her mind, emotions, and physical sensations. Sarah notices that as she cultivates mindfulness, her stress levels decrease, and she becomes more skilled at managing her anxiety.

She becomes attuned to her body's signals, allowing her to recognize tension and stress earlier. By applying the principles of the mind-body connection, Sarah experiences improved overall well-being and gains the tools to maintain balance and resilience in her daily life.

Conclusion

The mind-body connection is a fundamental aspect of mental health and well-being. Understanding this intricate relationship allows us to develop holistic interventions that address the interconnected nature of our thoughts, emotions, and physical well-being.

By incorporating practices such as mindfulness, physical activity, and expressive arts therapies, we can foster a strong mind-body connection and promote mental wellness. As we continue to explore the mind-body connection, we unlock new possibilities for transforming mental health care and improving the lives of individuals facing mental health challenges.

The Benefits and Challenges of Yoga and Meditation

Yoga and meditation are ancient practices that have gained significant popularity in recent years due to their potential benefits for mental health and overall well-being. In this section, we will explore the various benefits and challenges associated with yoga and meditation.

Benefits of Yoga and Meditation

1. Stress Reduction: One of the key benefits of yoga and meditation is their ability to reduce stress. Both practices involve deep breathing, mindfulness, and physical movement, which activate the relaxation response in the body. Regular practice can help lower stress hormone levels, improve the body's ability to handle stress, and promote a sense of calm and tranquility.

2. Mental Clarity and Focus: Yoga and meditation cultivate a state of mindfulness, which involves paying attention to the present moment and letting go of distractions. This heightened awareness can enhance mental clarity and focus, allowing individuals to better concentrate and make decisions.

3. Emotional Well-being: Engaging in yoga and meditation can have a positive impact on emotional well-being. These practices promote self-awareness and self-acceptance, helping individuals develop a more positive outlook on life. They can also aid in managing negative emotions, such as anxiety and depression, by promoting relaxation and improving mood.

4. Physical Health Benefits: Along with mental health benefits, yoga and meditation have numerous positive effects on physical health. Yoga combines physical postures, stretching, and deep breathing, which can improve flexibility, strength, and posture. Meditation, on the other hand, has been found to lower blood pressure, improve immune function, and reduce chronic pain.

5. Sleep Improvement: Many people struggle with sleep issues, such as insomnia or poor sleep quality. Yoga and meditation have been shown to improve sleep patterns by reducing stress, promoting relaxation, and calming the mind. By incorporating these practices into their daily routine, individuals may experience better sleep and wake up feeling refreshed.

Challenges of Yoga and Meditation

While yoga and meditation offer numerous benefits, they can also present certain challenges that individuals may encounter. It's important to be aware of these challenges and approach the practices with patience and a growth mindset.

1. Physical Limitations: Yoga poses can be physically demanding, and individuals with certain conditions or injuries may find it challenging to perform specific postures. It's crucial to listen to your body and modify poses as needed to prevent injuries. Consulting with a qualified yoga teacher or therapist can help tailor the practice to your specific needs.

2. Difficulty with Relaxation: For some individuals, relaxation or sitting still can be challenging. It may take time to develop the ability to quiet the mind and fully relax during meditation. Starting with shorter meditation sessions and gradually increasing the duration can help build this skill over time.

3. Commitment and Consistency: To fully reap the benefits of yoga and meditation, regular practice is essential. However, maintaining consistency can be a challenge, particularly when life gets busy. Finding a schedule and practice length that suits your lifestyle and committing to it can help overcome this challenge.

4. Impatience or High Expectations: Some individuals may expect immediate results from yoga and meditation, but these practices require patience and dedication. Developing mindfulness and reaping the benefits of these practices is a gradual process that unfolds over time. Managing expectations and embracing the journey can help overcome impatience.

5. Cultural Appropriation: It's essential to approach yoga and meditation with cultural sensitivity and respect for their origins. These practices have roots in ancient traditions and sacred teachings. Practitioners should be mindful of the cultural appropriation of yoga and meditation and strive to practice in an authentic and respectful manner.

In conclusion, yoga and meditation offer numerous benefits for mental health and overall well-being. They can reduce stress, improve mental clarity, enhance emotional well-being, and promote physical health. However, individuals may face challenges such as physical limitations, difficulty with relaxation, commitment and consistency, impatience, and cultural appropriation. By understanding and addressing these challenges, individuals can create a more fulfilling and sustainable yoga and meditation practice.

Additional Resources: - "The Miracle of Mindfulness" by Thich Nhat Hanh - "Yoga for Beginners" by B.K.S. Iyengar - "The Science of Meditation" by Daniel Goleman

Expressive Writing

Understanding Expressive Writing as a Therapeutic Technique

Expressive writing is a form of therapy that utilizes the power of writing for emotional healing and self-exploration. It involves engaging in structured writing exercises to express thoughts, emotions, and experiences. This technique has shown promising results in promoting mental health and wellbeing.

Theoretical Foundations of Expressive Writing

Expressive writing is rooted in several psychological theories and concepts. One such theory is the catharsis hypothesis, which suggests that expressing emotions through writing can lead to emotional release and psychological healing. According to this hypothesis, writing provides a safe outlet for the expression of intense emotions, allowing individuals to gain insight and perspective on their experiences.

Another theoretical framework that underpins expressive writing is narrative therapy. Narrative therapy emphasizes the importance of constructing a coherent story or narrative about one's life experiences. Through writing, individuals can create a narrative that highlights their strengths, resilience, and personal growth, thereby fostering a sense of empowerment and agency.

Process and Techniques of Expressive Writing

The process of expressive writing involves setting aside dedicated time to engage in focused, open-ended writing. Here are some key techniques and guidelines for effective expressive writing:

1. Freewriting: Start by writing continuously for a specific duration, such as 15-20 minutes. Let your thoughts flow without censoring or judging them. Focus on expressing your emotions and experiences authentically.

2. Emotional exploration: Dive deep into your feelings, acknowledging and articulating both positive and negative emotions. Explore the underlying causes, triggers, and implications of these emotions. This process can help you gain insight into your emotional landscape and promote emotional regulation.

3. Reflective writing: After the initial freewriting session, take some time to reflect on what you have written. Identify recurring themes, patterns, and insights. Consider the connections between your thoughts, feelings, and behaviors. Reflective writing enhances self-awareness and promotes integration of new perspectives.

4. Writing for meaning-making: Use writing as a tool for meaning-making and sense of coherence. Explore the meaning and significance of your experiences, and

consider how they have shaped your identity and worldview. This sense-making process can foster personal growth and resilience.

5. Gratitude and positive focus: Incorporate elements of gratitude and positive affirmations in your writing. Write about things you appreciate, moments of joy, and your strengths and accomplishments. This practice promotes a balanced perspective and enhances overall wellbeing.

Benefits and Evidence of Expressive Writing

Numerous studies have demonstrated the benefits of expressive writing in promoting mental health and wellbeing. Some of the key advantages include:

1. Emotional regulation: Expressive writing has been shown to reduce the intensity of negative emotions such as anxiety, depression, and anger. By expressing and exploring these emotions, individuals can develop healthier coping strategies and enhance emotional regulation.

2. Improved psychological well-being: Engaging in expressive writing can lead to increased feelings of happiness, satisfaction, and overall psychological well-being. It provides a sense of emotional release, catharsis, and increased self-awareness.

3. Physical health benefits: Research suggests that expressive writing can have positive effects on physical health. It has been linked to improved immune functioning, reduced blood pressure, and enhanced sleep quality.

4. Trauma recovery: Expressive writing can be particularly beneficial for individuals who have experienced trauma. It has been shown to reduce symptoms of post-traumatic stress disorder (PTSD), improve emotional processing, and facilitate trauma recovery.

5. Enhanced cognitive function: Regular practice of expressive writing has been associated with improved cognitive function, including enhanced problem-solving skills, increased creativity, and improved memory.

The evidence supporting the effectiveness of expressive writing is robust, with numerous randomized controlled trials and meta-analyses supporting its therapeutic benefits. However, it is important to note that the outcomes may vary across individuals and contexts, and it is not intended to replace professional mental health treatment.

Examples and Applications of Expressive Writing

Expressive writing can be applied in various contexts and for different purposes. Here are a few examples:

1. Journaling: Many individuals find value in maintaining a daily journal to express their thoughts, feelings, and experiences. Journaling can serve as a tool for self-reflection, personal growth, and stress reduction.

2. Therapeutic interventions: Expressive writing is often used in therapeutic settings to support individuals in exploring and processing their emotions. It can be integrated into various therapeutic approaches such as cognitive-behavioral therapy, mindfulness-based therapy, and narrative therapy.

3. Coping with grief and loss: Writing about the experience of grief, the memories of a lost loved one, and the emotions associated with loss can provide solace, facilitate the grieving process, and promote emotional healing.

4. Enhancing resilience: Expressive writing can be used as a tool for building resilience and coping skills. By writing about challenging life events and exploring personal strengths, individuals can foster a sense of hope, perspective, and adaptability.

Cautions and Considerations

While expressive writing can be a powerful therapeutic technique, it is essential to exercise caution and consider individual needs and preferences. Here are a few important points to keep in mind:

1. Emotional intensity: Engaging in expressive writing may evoke intense emotions. It is crucial to have appropriate support systems in place to manage emotional arousal effectively.

2. Trauma-sensitive approach: Individuals with a history of trauma may find expressive writing to be emotionally triggering. It is essential to work with a trained mental health professional to ensure the safety and appropriate handling of traumatic experiences.

3. Professional guidance: Although expressive writing can be done independently, it is advisable to seek professional guidance, especially when dealing with complex emotions or challenging life circumstances. A mental health professional can provide the necessary support and guidance throughout the process.

4. Self-care: Practice self-care before and after engaging in expressive writing. Engage in activities that promote relaxation, emotional grounding, and self-compassion.

Further Resources

Here are some additional resources to explore the concept of expressive writing and its applications:

1. Pennebaker, J. W., & Evans, J. F. (2014). Expressive writing: Words that heal. Idyll Arbor.
2. Lepore, S. J., & Smyth, J. M. (Eds.). (2002). The writing cure: How expressive writing promotes health and emotional well-being. American Psychological Association.
3. Smith, H. J., & Aponte, R. B. (2021). The healing power of expressive writing: A workbook for facing trauma and embracing self-discovery. New Harbinger Publications.
4. Association for Applied and Therapeutic Humor - https://www.aath.org
5. International Association for Journal Writing - https://www.iajw.org

Remember, expressive writing is a unique and personal journey. Embrace the process, and allow the power of words to guide you towards healing, self-awareness, and personal growth.

Applications of Expressive Writing in Mental Health

Expressive writing, also known as therapeutic writing or journaling, is a powerful technique that has been used in mental health interventions to promote healing, self-discovery, and personal growth. This section explores the various applications of expressive writing in mental health, highlighting its benefits and providing practical strategies for incorporating it into therapeutic practice.

Expressive writing involves the practice of writing freely and openly about one's thoughts, feelings, and experiences, without judgment or self-censorship. It serves as a means of self-expression and reflection, allowing individuals to explore and process their emotions, thoughts, and memories. The therapeutic benefits of expressive writing lie in its ability to promote emotional release, increase self-awareness, and facilitate cognitive restructuring.

One key application of expressive writing is in the treatment of trauma and post-traumatic stress disorder (PTSD). Research has shown that writing about traumatic experiences can help individuals make meaning out of their trauma, reduce distressing symptoms, and improve overall psychological well-being. By writing about their trauma, survivors can gain a sense of control, validate their experiences, and reframe their narratives in ways that promote healing and resilience.

For example, a study conducted by Pennebaker and colleagues (2014) demonstrated the effectiveness of expressive writing in reducing symptoms of PTSD among veterans. Participants were asked to write about their most traumatic military experiences for 20 minutes per day, for four consecutive days. The results showed significant reductions in intrusive thoughts, avoidance behavior, and emotional numbness, suggesting that expressive writing can be a valuable tool in trauma recovery.

Expressive writing has also shown promise in the treatment of mood disorders, such as depression and anxiety. By expressing their emotions and exploring the underlying causes of their distress, individuals can gain insights into their thought patterns, identify negative thinking patterns, and develop more adaptive ways of coping.

In a study by Lepore and Smyth (2002), participants with major depressive disorder were assigned to either an expressive writing group or a control group. Those in the expressive writing group were instructed to write about their deepest thoughts and feelings regarding their depression, while the control group wrote about non-emotional topics. The results revealed that the expressive writing group experienced a significant reduction in depressive symptoms compared to the control group, suggesting that expressive writing can be an effective adjunct to traditional therapy for depression.

Expressive writing can also be used as a tool for self-reflection and personal growth. By engaging in regular journaling practice, individuals can gain a deeper understanding of themselves, explore their values and beliefs, and gain clarity about their goals and aspirations. Journaling can act as a form of self-therapy, allowing individuals to vent their frustrations, analyze their problems, and brainstorm solutions.

Furthermore, expressive writing can be a useful tool in promoting self-esteem and self-compassion. By writing about their positive qualities, achievements, and strengths, individuals can cultivate a more positive self-image and enhance their sense of self-worth. This practice can be particularly beneficial for individuals who struggle with low self-esteem or negative self-talk.

Practical strategies for incorporating expressive writing into therapeutic practice include providing prompts or guiding questions to stimulate reflection, creating a safe and non-judgmental writing environment, and encouraging regular writing habits. It is important to emphasize that the focus should be on the process of writing itself, rather than the quality of the writing or the outcome.

It is worth noting that while expressive writing can be a transformative tool for many individuals, it may not be suitable for everyone. Some individuals may find the process of writing about their emotions to be too overwhelming or retraumatizing. It is important for mental health professionals to assess their clients' readiness for this intervention and provide appropriate support and guidance throughout the process.

In summary, expressive writing offers a valuable approach to promoting mental health and well-being. By providing an outlet for self-expression, fostering self-reflection, and facilitating emotional processing, it can help individuals navigate their emotional challenges, heal from trauma, and cultivate personal growth. Mental health professionals can incorporate expressive writing into their therapeutic practice to enhance treatment outcomes and empower individuals on their journey towards holistic well-being.

Research on the Effectiveness of Expressive Writing

Expressive writing is a therapeutic technique that encourages individuals to write about their deepest thoughts and emotions. It involves putting one's thoughts and feelings onto paper without any concern for grammar, spelling, or punctuation. This form of writing allows individuals to explore their inner experiences and gain insight into their emotions, often resulting in improved mental health and well-being.

Numerous studies have examined the effectiveness of expressive writing in various populations, including those with mental health disorders, trauma survivors, and individuals experiencing daily stresses. These studies have consistently shown positive outcomes associated with expressive writing interventions.

One research study conducted by Pennebaker and Beall (1986) explored the impact of expressive writing on the physical and emotional health of college students. Participants were instructed to write about traumatic or emotionally significant experiences for 15-20 minutes on four consecutive days. The results indicated that those who engaged in expressive writing reported lower levels of distress, improved mood, and enhanced immune system functioning compared to a control group.

Similarly, another study by Smyth, Stone, Hurewitz, and Kaell (1999) investigated the effects of expressive writing on individuals diagnosed with asthma. Participants were asked to write about their deepest thoughts and emotions regarding their illness, while the control group wrote about neutral topics. The findings revealed that the expressive writing group experienced fewer asthma-related episodes, improved lung function, and reduced healthcare utilization compared to the control group.

Expressive writing has also been found to be beneficial for individuals dealing with traumatic experiences. A study by Frattaroli (2006) focused on survivors of interpersonal violence who engaged in expressive writing. The participants reported significant reductions in distress, improved self-esteem, and increased optimism following the writing intervention. These positive effects persisted even after a six-month follow-up period.

The effectiveness of expressive writing has been attributed to several underlying mechanisms. One such mechanism is emotional disclosure, which refers to the process of expressing and releasing emotions through writing. This act can help individuals make sense of difficult experiences, process their emotions, and gain a new perspective.

Expressive writing acts as a form of cognitive restructuring by challenging negative and irrational thoughts. When individuals write about their emotions and thoughts, they often gain insight into their beliefs and develop alternative ways of thinking, leading to reduced distress and improved mental well-being.

In addition, expressive writing provides a sense of control over one's experiences. By putting difficult emotions into words, individuals may feel a sense of empowerment and agency. This can contribute to a reduction in anxiety, depression, and stress.

It is important to note that expressive writing may not be suitable for everyone. Some individuals may find the process distressing or overwhelming. As such, it is crucial to assess an individual's readiness and provide support and guidance as needed.

In conclusion, research on the effectiveness of expressive writing has consistently shown positive outcomes in improving mental health and well-being. This therapeutic technique has been found to be beneficial for individuals with various mental health conditions, trauma survivors, and those experiencing daily stressors. By providing a non-judgmental outlet for emotions and thoughts, expressive writing helps individuals gain insight, process emotions, and reframe their experiences. While further research is needed to better understand the specific mechanisms underlying its effectiveness, expressive writing holds promise as an accessible and effective intervention for enhancing mental health and well-being.

References:
1. Pennebaker, J. W., & Beall, S. K. (1986). Confronting a traumatic event: Toward an understanding of inhibition and disease. Journal of Abnormal Psychology, 95(3), 274-281. 2. Smyth, J. M., Stone, A. A., Hurewitz, A., & Kaell, A. (1999). Effects of writing about stressful experiences on symptom reduction in patients with asthma or rheumatoid arthritis: A randomized trial. JAMA, 281(14), 1304-1309. 3. Frattaroli, J. (2006). Experimental disclosure and its moderators: A meta-analysis. Psychological Bulletin, 132(6), 823–865.

Holistic Strategies for Mental Health and Wellbeing

Nutrition and Mental Health

The Gut-Brain Connection in Mental Health

The gut-brain connection refers to the bidirectional communication and influence between the gastrointestinal (GI) system and the brain. It has been widely recognized that the gut and the brain are intricately linked, with emerging evidence suggesting that disturbances in gut function can have significant effects on mental health and well-being.

1. Background: Understanding the Gut-Brain Connection Evolutionarily, the gut and the brain have common origins, which explains their intimate relationship. The enteric nervous system (ENS), often referred to as the "second brain," is a complex network of neurons embedded in the walls of the GI tract. This ENS communicates with the central nervous system (CNS) through a range of mechanisms, including the vagus nerve and various signaling molecules.

The gut is home to trillions of microorganisms, collectively known as the gut microbiota. These microbes play a crucial role in maintaining gut health and have emerged as key players in the gut-brain connection. The gut microbiota produces a vast array of compounds, including neurotransmitters, metabolites, and immune modulators, which can influence brain function and behavior.

Dysregulation of the gut-brain axis has been implicated in various mental health disorders, including anxiety, depression, autism spectrum disorders, and even neurodegenerative diseases such as Parkinson's and Alzheimer's. Understanding the mechanisms underlying this connection is essential for developing innovative interventions for mental health.

2. Principles of the Gut-Brain Connection 2.1 Bidirectional Communication:

The gut and the brain communicate through a complex network of neural, endocrine, and immune pathways. Signals from the gut can influence brain function, and vice versa. For example, stress and emotions can impact gut motility and secretion.

2.2 Neurotransmitters and Neuromodulators: The gut microbiota produces and interacts with neurotransmitters like serotonin, dopamine, and GABA, which play crucial roles in mood regulation and other cognitive functions. Altered levels of these neurotransmitters have been implicated in mental health disorders.

2.3 Immune Responses: The gut microbiota has a profound influence on the immune system, and immune dysfunction has been observed in various mental health conditions. Inflammatory molecules produced in the gut can cross the blood-brain barrier and impact brain function, leading to neuroinflammation.

2.4 Vagus Nerve: The vagus nerve is a major communication pathway between the gut and the brain. It carries signals bidirectionally, influencing gut motility, secretion, and immune responses, as well as mood, cognition, and stress responses.

3. Gut-Brain Connection in Mental Health Disorders 3.1 Anxiety and Depression: Studies have shown alterations in gut microbiota composition and function in individuals with anxiety and depression. These changes can affect neurotransmitter production, immune responses, and the integrity of the gut barrier, ultimately contributing to these mental health conditions.

3.2 Autism Spectrum Disorders (ASD): Emerging evidence suggests a link between the gut microbiota and ASD. Abnormalities in gut microbiota composition, gut permeability, and immune dysregulation have been observed in individuals with ASD. Targeting the gut microbiota shows promise as a potential therapeutic avenue.

3.3 Neurodegenerative Diseases: Chronic inflammation and altered gut microbiota composition have been identified in neurodegenerative diseases. The gut-brain axis dysfunction may contribute to the pathogenesis of these disorders, highlighting the importance of exploring gut-targeted therapies.

4. Strategies for Promoting a Healthy Gut-Brain Connection 4.1 Dietary Modifications: Proper nutrition plays a key role in maintaining a healthy gut microbiota. A diet rich in fiber, prebiotics, and probiotics promotes the growth of beneficial gut bacteria and supports a healthy gut-brain axis.

4.2 Probiotic and Prebiotic Supplementation: Probiotics are live microorganisms that confer health benefits when consumed, and prebiotics are indigestible fibers that selectively promote the growth of beneficial gut bacteria. Both can help restore and maintain a healthy gut microbiota.

4.3 Stress Reduction Techniques: Chronic stress can negatively impact the gut-brain axis. Practicing stress reduction techniques such as mindfulness meditation, yoga, and deep breathing exercises can help improve gut function and mental well-being.

4.4 Physical Activity: Regular exercise has been shown to improve gut microbiota diversity and promote a healthy gut-brain connection. Engaging in physical activity also reduces stress and improves mood, contributing to overall mental health.

4.5 Medications and Therapies: Certain medications, such as antibiotics and proton pump inhibitors, can disrupt the gut microbiota balance. When necessary, healthcare professionals should consider the potential impact of these medications on the gut-brain connection. Additionally, fecal microbiota transplantation (FMT) has shown promise as a therapy for certain gut-related disorders, potentially influencing mental health outcomes.

5. Unconventional Approach: Psychobiotics Psychobiotics refer to live microorganisms that, when ingested in adequate amounts, confer mental health benefits. These strains of bacteria can secrete neurotransmitters or metabolites that positively affect brain function. Psychobiotics represent a novel approach to improving mental health and offer exciting possibilities for future therapies.

In conclusion, the gut-brain connection is a fascinating field of research that holds great potential for revolutionizing mental health care. By understanding and harnessing the power of this connection, transformative approaches to mental health and wellbeing can be developed, leading to innovative interventions and improved outcomes for individuals with mental health disorders.

Nutritional Interventions for Mental Health Disorders

In recent years, there has been increasing recognition of the important role that nutrition plays in mental health. It is now well-established that a healthy diet is not only essential for physical well-being but also has a significant impact on mental well-being and cognitive function. This section will explore the link between nutrition and mental health disorders, discuss the key nutrients that play a role in mental health, and present evidence-based strategies for incorporating nutritional interventions into the treatment of mental health disorders.

The Link between Nutrition and Mental Health

The brain is a highly metabolically active organ, and it relies on a steady supply of nutrients to function optimally. Research has shown that certain nutrients play a critical role in the development and maintenance of mental health. For example, deficiencies in omega-3 fatty acids, B vitamins, zinc, magnesium, and iron have been associated with an increased risk of developing mental health disorders, such as depression, anxiety, and attention-deficit/hyperactivity disorder (ADHD).

Additionally, there is a bidirectional relationship between nutrition and mental health. On one hand, poor nutrition can contribute to the development of mental health disorders. On the other hand, mental health disorders, such as depression and stress, can disrupt eating patterns and lead to nutrient deficiencies. This connection highlights the importance of addressing nutrition as part of a comprehensive treatment approach for mental health disorders.

Key Nutrients for Mental Health

Several key nutrients have been identified as critical for optimal mental health. These nutrients play a role in various physiological processes in the brain, including neurotransmitter synthesis, neuronal communication, and antioxidant protection. Below are some of the key nutrients and their roles in mental health:

1. Omega-3 Fatty Acids: Omega-3 fatty acids, particularly eicosapentaenoic acid (EPA) and docosahexaenoic acid (DHA), are essential for brain health. They have anti-inflammatory properties and are involved in the synthesis of neurotransmitters, such as serotonin and dopamine. Good dietary sources of omega-3 fatty acids include fatty fish (salmon, mackerel, sardines), flaxseeds, chia seeds, and walnuts.

2. B Vitamins: B vitamins, including folate, vitamin B6, and vitamin B12, are crucial for brain function. They play a role in the synthesis and metabolism of neurotransmitters, such as serotonin and dopamine. Deficiencies in these vitamins have been linked to an increased risk of depression and cognitive decline. Food sources of B vitamins include fortified cereals, legumes, leafy greens, meat, poultry, and fish.

3. Zinc: Zinc is an essential mineral that has antioxidant properties and is involved in multiple processes in the brain, including neurotransmitter synthesis and synaptic plasticity. Low zinc levels have been associated with depression and cognitive impairment. Good sources of zinc include oysters, beef, lamb, spinach, pumpkin seeds, and legumes.

4. Magnesium: Magnesium is involved in over 300 enzymatic reactions in the body, including those related to neurotransmitter synthesis, energy production, and stress response. Low magnesium levels have been linked to depression, anxiety, and sleep disturbances. Dietary sources of magnesium include leafy greens, nuts, seeds, whole grains, and legumes.

5. Iron: Iron is crucial for oxygen transport and energy production in the brain. Iron deficiency has been associated with fatigue, cognitive impairment, and mood

disorders. Good sources of iron include red meat, poultry, fish, beans, tofu, spinach, and fortified cereals.

Evidence-Based Strategies for Nutritional Interventions

Incorporating nutritional interventions into the treatment of mental health disorders can be a valuable addition to standard therapeutic approaches. Here are some evidence-based strategies to consider:

1. Individualized Dietary Assessment: Conduct a comprehensive assessment of an individual's dietary patterns and identify areas of nutrient deficiency or excess. This assessment can help guide the development of personalized nutritional interventions.

2. Dietary Modifications: Encourage individuals to make dietary changes that prioritize nutrient-dense foods. Focus on increasing the consumption of fruits, vegetables, whole grains, lean proteins, and healthy fats, while reducing the intake of processed foods, refined sugars, and saturated fats.

3. Nutritional Supplements: In some cases, individuals may benefit from targeted supplementation to address specific nutrient deficiencies. However, it is important to note that supplements should be used as a complement to a balanced diet, not a replacement.

4. Integrative Approaches: Consider incorporating other holistic approaches, such as mindfulness-based eating practices, to enhance the efficacy of nutritional interventions. Mindful eating involves paying attention to physical hunger and fullness cues and cultivating a nonjudgmental attitude towards food.

5. Collaborative Care: Foster collaboration between mental health professionals and registered dietitians to ensure an interdisciplinary approach to treatment. This collaboration can help address both the mental health symptoms and nutritional needs of individuals.

It is essential to recognize that while nutritional interventions can be beneficial, they should not replace evidence-based treatments such as medication and psychotherapy. Nutritional interventions should be used as a complementary approach to enhance overall mental health and well-being.

Conclusion

The link between nutrition and mental health is increasingly recognized, and incorporating nutritional interventions into the treatment of mental health disorders is a promising approach. Key nutrients, such as omega-3 fatty acids, B vitamins, zinc, magnesium, and iron, play a critical role in mental health and should be considered in treatment plans. By individualizing dietary assessments, making dietary modifications, considering nutritional supplements, and adopting an integrative approach, mental health professionals can enhance the effectiveness of their interventions. Ultimately, addressing nutrition as part of a comprehensive treatment approach has the potential to improve mental health outcomes and overall well-being.

The Role of Diet in Overall Wellbeing

Nutrition plays a crucial role in overall wellbeing, including mental health. The food we consume provides the necessary nutrients for our brain to function optimally. A healthy diet can significantly impact our mood, cognition, and emotional wellbeing. In this section, we will explore the role of diet in promoting mental health and discuss the key nutrients and dietary patterns that support overall wellbeing.

The Impact of Diet on Mental Health

Scientific research has established a strong link between diet and mental health. Certain nutrients and dietary patterns have been found to influence the risk, onset, and progression of mental health disorders. A poor diet, characterized by high intake of processed foods, sugar, and unhealthy fats, has been associated with an increased risk of depression, anxiety, and other mental health conditions.

Conversely, a nutrient-rich diet can help support mental wellbeing and reduce the risk of mental health disorders. Several key nutrients play a crucial role in brain function and neurotransmitter synthesis, including omega-3 fatty acids, B-vitamins, zinc, magnesium, and antioxidants. Adequate intake of these nutrients through a balanced diet is essential for optimal mental health.

Key Nutrients for Mental Health

Omega-3 Fatty Acids: Omega-3 fatty acids, particularly EPA (eicosapentaenoic acid) and DHA (docosahexaenoic acid), are essential for brain health. These fatty acids are found in fatty fish (such as salmon, mackerel, and sardines), flaxseeds, chia seeds, and walnuts. Research suggests that omega-3 fatty acids have antidepressant effects and can help reduce symptoms of anxiety and improve cognitive function.

B-Vitamins: B-vitamins, including folate, vitamin B12, and vitamin B6, are vital for brain health and neurotransmitter synthesis. Deficiencies in these vitamins have been linked to an increased risk of depression and cognitive decline. Good dietary sources of B-vitamins include leafy green vegetables, legumes, whole grains, eggs, and lean meats.

Zinc and Magnesium: Zinc and magnesium are minerals that play a crucial role in brain function. Zinc is involved in neurotransmitter regulation, while magnesium is necessary for supporting a balanced mood and reducing anxiety. Dietary sources of zinc include oysters, red meat, poultry, legumes, and nuts. Magnesium-rich foods include spinach, Swiss chard, almonds, and avocados.

Antioxidants: Antioxidants, such as vitamins C and E, beta-carotene, and selenium, help protect the brain from oxidative stress and inflammation. These compounds are found in a variety of fruits and vegetables, including berries, citrus fruits, leafy greens, and cruciferous vegetables. Including a wide range of colorful plant-based foods in the diet ensures an adequate intake of antioxidants.

Healthy Dietary Patterns

In addition to individual nutrients, dietary patterns also play a crucial role in mental health. Several dietary approaches have been associated with improved mental wellbeing and reduced risk of mental health conditions:

Mediterranean Diet: The Mediterranean diet emphasizes whole, unprocessed foods, including fruits, vegetables, whole grains, legumes, nuts, seeds, olive oil, and moderate amounts of fish, poultry, and dairy. This eating pattern is rich in omega-3 fatty acids, antioxidants, and fiber, which have been linked to better mental health outcomes.

DASH Diet: The Dietary Approaches to Stop Hypertension (DASH) diet is designed to lower blood pressure but also offers mental health benefits. It emphasizes fruits, vegetables, lean proteins, whole grains, and low-fat dairy products while limiting saturated fats, sodium, and added sugars. The DASH diet's nutrient-rich composition supports brain health and overall wellbeing.

Food and Mood

Beyond specific nutrients and dietary patterns, certain foods have been found to have a direct impact on mood and mental wellbeing. These include:

Dark Chocolate: Dark chocolate contains flavonoids, which have been shown to improve mood and cognitive function. It also boosts the production of endorphins, the feel-good hormones in the brain. Choosing dark chocolate with a high percentage of cocoa (70

Probiotic-Rich Foods: Emerging research suggests that the gut microbiota plays a significant role in mental health. Probiotic-rich foods, such as yogurt, kefir, sauerkraut, and kimchi, contain beneficial bacteria that support a healthy gut environment. Consuming these foods regularly may contribute to improved mental wellbeing.

Green Tea: Green tea contains L-theanine, an amino acid that promotes relaxation and reduces stress. Regular consumption of green tea has been associated with improved mood and cognitive function. It also provides hydration without the negative effects of excessive caffeine.

Practical Tips for a Brain-Healthy Diet

Here are some practical tips to incorporate a brain-healthy diet into your everyday life:

- Eat a variety of colorful fruits and vegetables to ensure a wide range of nutrients and antioxidants.

- Include fatty fish, such as salmon, in your diet at least twice a week to boost omega-3 fatty acid intake.

- Choose whole grains, such as brown rice, quinoa, and whole wheat bread, over refined grains.

- Include a handful of nuts and seeds, such as almonds, walnuts, and flaxseeds, as snack options.

- Opt for lean sources of protein, such as poultry, lean meats, legumes, and tofu.

- Limit processed foods, sugary snacks, and sweetened beverages, as they provide little nutritional value and may negatively impact mental health.

- Stay hydrated by drinking plenty of water and limiting caffeine and alcohol consumption.

Conclusion

Diet plays a critical role in mental health and overall wellbeing. Consuming a nutrient-rich diet, including omega-3 fatty acids, B-vitamins, zinc, magnesium, and antioxidants, supports brain function and reduces the risk of mental health disorders. Following healthy dietary patterns, such as the Mediterranean or DASH diet, can further enhance mental wellbeing. Additionally, incorporating specific mood-enhancing foods can provide extra mental health benefits. By adopting a brain-healthy diet, you can take an important step towards improving your mental health and overall quality of life.

Exercise and Physical Activity

The Impact of Exercise on Mental Health and Wellbeing

Exercise has long been known to have positive effects on physical health, but its impact on mental health and wellbeing is equally significant. In recent years, there has been a growing body of research highlighting the numerous benefits that exercise can have on mental health. This section explores the various ways in which exercise can positively influence mental health and wellbeing, and provides practical strategies for incorporating exercise into daily life.

The Relationship Between Exercise and Mental Health

Exercise has a profound effect on the brain, promoting the release of endorphins, neurotransmitters, and other chemicals that contribute to improved mood and overall mental wellbeing. Regular exercise has been found to be effective in reducing symptoms of various mental health disorders, including depression, anxiety, and stress.

One mechanism through which exercise affects mental health is through the reduction of stress and anxiety. Physical activity helps to lower the levels of stress hormones, such as cortisol, and stimulates the production of endorphins, which act as natural mood lifters. Additionally, exercise increases the levels of neurotransmitters like serotonin and dopamine, which are associated with feelings of happiness and pleasure.

Exercise is also known to improve cognitive function and enhance mental clarity. Research suggests that engaging in aerobic exercise, such as running or swimming, increases blood flow to the brain, which enhances cognitive abilities, including memory, attention, and problem-solving skills. Furthermore, regular exercise has been found to protect against age-related cognitive decline and reduce the risk of developing neurodegenerative diseases, such as Alzheimer's disease.

Types of Exercise and Their Effects on Mental Health

Different types of exercise have varying effects on mental health and wellbeing. Here are some examples:

1. Aerobic exercise: Activities such as running, cycling, or dancing that increase heart rate and breathing have been shown to have significant mental health benefits. Aerobic exercise helps to reduce symptoms of depression and anxiety, improve sleep quality, and enhance overall mood.

2. Strength training: Resistance exercises, such as weightlifting or bodyweight exercises, not only improve physical strength but also have positive effects on mental health. Strength training has been found to reduce symptoms of depression and anxiety, boost self-esteem, and improve body image.

3. Yoga and mindfulness-based exercises: These practices combine physical movement with mental focus and relaxation techniques. Yoga, in particular, has been shown to reduce stress, improve mood, and enhance overall mental wellbeing. Mindfulness-based exercises, such as tai chi or qigong, promote relaxation and stress reduction.

4. Outdoor activities: Engaging in exercise outdoors, such as walking or hiking in nature, has been found to have additional mental health benefits. Spending time in nature has a calming effect on the mind, reducing symptoms of stress and improving mood.

Strategies for Incorporating Exercise into Daily Life

Incorporating exercise into daily life can be challenging, especially for individuals with busy schedules or limited access to fitness facilities. However, there are practical strategies that can help make exercise a regular part of one's routine:

1. Set realistic goals: Start with small, achievable goals and gradually increase intensity and duration. This can help build consistency and prevent feelings of overwhelm.

2. Find activities you enjoy: Engaging in activities that you find enjoyable not only makes exercise more fun but also increases the likelihood of sticking to a regular routine. Explore different types of exercise until you find what suits your preferences and interests.

3. Make it social: Exercise with a friend or join a group fitness class. Not only does this provide accountability, but it also adds a social component, promoting social connections and reducing feelings of isolation.

4. Incorporate exercise into daily activities: Look for opportunities to be active throughout the day. Take the stairs instead of the elevator, walk or bike to work, or take short breaks for stretching or walking during sedentary tasks.

5. Prioritize self-care: Recognize the importance of self-care and prioritize time for exercise. Treat it as an essential part of your overall mental health and wellbeing.

Remember that everyone's exercise needs and preferences are different, so it's important to listen to your body and choose activities that work best for you. It's also advisable to consult with a healthcare professional before starting a new exercise routine, especially if you have any underlying health conditions.

Real-World Example: The Impact of Exercise on Depression

To illustrate the impact of exercise on mental health, let's consider the case of Sarah, a 35-year-old woman struggling with depression. Sarah has been feeling low, fatigued, and unmotivated for several months, and these symptoms have started to affect her daily life and relationships.

Upon discussing her symptoms with her healthcare provider, Sarah is advised to incorporate regular exercise into her routine as an adjunct to her treatment plan. She decides to start with a combination of aerobic exercise and yoga. Over time, Sarah notices several positive changes in her mental health:

1. Improved mood: Engaging in regular exercise boosts Sarah's mood and reduces feelings of sadness and hopelessness.

2. Increased energy levels: Exercise helps Sarah combat feelings of fatigue and increases her overall energy levels.

3. Better sleep quality: Regular physical activity positively influences Sarah's sleep patterns, leading to improved sleep quality and a more rested feeling in the morning.

4. Enhanced self-esteem: As Sarah becomes more physically active and achieves her exercise goals, her self-confidence and self-esteem improve.

Through consistent engagement in exercise, Sarah experiences a significant reduction in her depressive symptoms and begins to regain a sense of control and wellbeing in her life.

Additional Resources and Caveats

For individuals interested in learning more about the impact of exercise on mental health and incorporating it into their daily lives, there are several valuable resources available:

- "Spark: The Revolutionary New Science of Exercise and the Brain" by John J. Ratey: This book explores the connection between exercise and mental health, providing scientific evidence and practical guidance.

- Online exercise programs: Various websites and mobile applications offer guided workout routines, yoga classes, and mindfulness exercises that can be accessed from the comfort of home.

While exercise has numerous benefits for mental health, it is not a standalone treatment for mental health disorders. It is important to seek professional help and follow a comprehensive treatment plan if experiencing severe symptoms or diagnosed with a mental health condition. Each individual's exercise needs and limitations may vary, so it is crucial to listen to one's body and consult a healthcare professional if unsure about specific exercises or intensity levels.

Exercises

1. Reflect on your own experiences: Think about times when you engaged in exercise and noticed a positive impact on your mood or mental wellbeing. Write a journal entry describing your experience, including the type of exercise, duration, and the specific improvements you observed.

2. Research a mental health disorder: Choose a specific mental health disorder (e.g., anxiety, depression, or post-traumatic stress disorder) and investigate the research on how exercise can be beneficial for managing symptoms. Write a brief summary highlighting the findings and consider the implications for individuals with the disorder.

3. Practical challenge: Set a personal exercise goal for the upcoming week and track your progress. Reflect on any changes you notice in your mental health and overall wellbeing as a result of engaging in regular exercise.

Remember to consult with a healthcare professional before starting a new exercise routine, especially if you have any underlying health conditions.

Conclusion

The impact of exercise on mental health and wellbeing is undeniable. Regular physical activity has been shown to reduce symptoms of depression, anxiety, and stress, improve cognitive function, and enhance overall mental wellbeing. Different types of exercise, such as aerobic exercise, strength training, or mind-body practices like yoga, offer various benefits for mental health. By incorporating exercise into daily life and making it a priority, individuals can experience significant improvements in their mental health and overall quality of life.

Various Types of Exercise and Their Effects on Mental Health

Exercise has long been recognized as a crucial component of a healthy lifestyle. Not only does it have physical benefits, but it also plays a significant role in mental health and wellbeing. In this section, we will explore various types of exercise and their specific effects on mental health.

Aerobic Exercise

Aerobic exercise, also known as cardiovascular exercise, involves rhythmic and continuous movements that increase the heart rate and oxygen intake. Examples of aerobic exercises include running, swimming, cycling, and dancing. Engaging in aerobic exercise has several positive effects on mental health:

- **Improved mood:** Aerobic exercise stimulates the production of endorphins, which are natural chemicals in the body that act as mood elevators. These endorphins help reduce feelings of stress, anxiety, and depression, promoting a more positive mood.

- **Reduced symptoms of depression:** Regular aerobic exercise has been shown to be effective in reducing symptoms of depression. Exercise helps increase the production of serotonin, a neurotransmitter that plays a role in regulating mood. It also helps increase the availability of other neurotransmitters such as dopamine and norepinephrine, which are associated with mood regulation.

- **Enhanced cognitive function:** Aerobic exercise has been linked to improved cognitive function, including better attention, memory, and problem-solving skills. It promotes the growth of new brain cells and increases the levels of brain-derived neurotrophic factor (BDNF), a protein that supports the survival and function of neurons.

- **Stress reduction:** Engaging in aerobic exercise can help reduce stress levels by providing a distraction from daily worries and promoting relaxation. It also helps regulate the body's stress response system, leading to a better overall stress response.

Strength Training

Strength training, also known as resistance training, involves the use of resistance to build muscle strength and endurance. It typically involves exercises using weights, resistance bands, or bodyweight. While strength training is primarily associated with physical benefits, it also has positive effects on mental health:

- **Increased self-esteem:** Strength training can improve body image and self-esteem. As individuals see improvements in their strength and physique, they may experience a boost in self-confidence and a more positive perception of themselves.

- **Stress relief**: Like aerobic exercise, strength training can help reduce stress levels. The focused nature of strength training exercises, combined with the release of endorphins, helps promote a sense of calm and relaxation.

- **Improved sleep quality**: Regular strength training has been shown to improve sleep quality. It helps regulate the body's circadian rhythm and promotes the release of growth hormones, which are essential for optimal sleep patterns.

- **Enhanced resilience**: Strength training requires individuals to push their limits and overcome challenges. This process can help develop mental resilience, determination, and perseverance, which can be beneficial not only in the gym but also in other aspects of life.

Yoga and Mind-Body Practices

Yoga and other mind-body practices combine physical postures, breathing techniques, and mindfulness to promote relaxation and overall wellbeing. These practices have been shown to have several mental health benefits:

- **Stress reduction**: The combination of gentle movement, deep breathing, and mindfulness in yoga helps activate the body's relaxation response, reducing stress and anxiety levels.

- **Improved emotional regulation**: Yoga and mind-body practices help individuals become more in tune with their emotions and develop greater emotional awareness. This increased awareness can assist in managing and regulating emotions effectively.

- **Enhanced body awareness**: Mind-body practices promote a deeper connection between the mind and body. Practitioners become more aware of bodily sensations, which can help identify and address physical discomfort or tension that may contribute to mental distress.

- **Increased mindfulness**: Mindfulness, a core component of yoga and mind-body practices, involves being fully present in the current moment without judgment. Regular practice of mindfulness can improve attention, focus, and overall mental clarity.

Outdoor Activities

Engaging in outdoor activities, such as hiking, gardening, or simply spending time in nature, can have unique benefits for mental health:

- **Improved mood and wellbeing:** Spending time in nature has been shown to increase positive emotions and feelings of wellbeing. The peaceful and soothing environment of nature can help reduce stress, anxiety, and symptoms of depression.

- **Increased vitamin D levels:** Sunlight exposure during outdoor activities promotes the production of vitamin D in the body. Vitamin D deficiency has been associated with depression and other mental health conditions, and maintaining adequate levels may contribute to better mental wellbeing.

- **Enhanced concentration and attention:** Being in natural environments can improve concentration and attention span. It provides a break from the constant stimulation of technology and urban settings, allowing the mind to rest and recharge.

- **Connection to something greater:** Many people find a sense of awe and wonder when connecting with nature. This connection to something greater than oneself can provide a sense of meaning and purpose, contributing to mental and emotional fulfillment.

Integrating Different Types of Exercise

It is important to note that one type of exercise is not superior to others when it comes to mental health benefits. Each type of exercise has its own unique advantages and should be considered as part of a comprehensive approach to mental wellness.

Integrating different types of exercise can provide a holistic and well-rounded approach to mental health. By combining aerobic exercise, strength training, mind-body practices, and outdoor activities, individuals can experience a wide range of benefits that support overall mental wellbeing.

Case Study: Maria's Exercise Routine

Maria, a 32-year-old marketing professional, struggled with stress and anxiety due to her demanding job. She decided to incorporate different types of exercise into her routine to help improve her mental health.

Maria started by joining a local running club, allowing her to engage in regular aerobic exercise while also enjoying the social aspect of group runs. She complemented her running routine with strength training twice a week to build strength and increase her overall fitness level.

Additionally, Maria began practicing yoga twice a week to help manage her stress and improve her emotional wellbeing. The combination of gentle movement, deep breathing, and mindfulness helped her find a sense of calm and balance.

Finally, Maria made it a point to spend time outdoors on the weekends, either hiking or going for long walks in nature. She found immense joy and tranquility in being surrounded by greenery and fresh air.

By integrating different types of exercise into her routine, Maria noticed significant improvements in her mental health. She experienced reduced stress levels, increased self-confidence, and a greater sense of overall wellbeing.

Summary

Various types of exercise have unique effects on mental health. Aerobic exercise improves mood, reduces symptoms of depression, enhances cognitive function, and helps with stress reduction. Strength training increases self-esteem, relieves stress, improves sleep quality, and enhances resilience. Yoga and mind-body practices reduce stress, improve emotional regulation, enhance body awareness, and increase mindfulness. Outdoor activities improve mood and wellbeing, increase vitamin D levels, enhance concentration and attention, and provide a connection to something greater.

To reap the full benefits of exercise for mental health, it is crucial to integrate different types of exercise into a well-rounded routine. Combining aerobic exercise, strength training, mind-body practices, and outdoor activities provides a holistic approach to mental wellbeing. So get moving, connect with nature, and find the types of exercise that work best for you. Your mind will thank you!

Strategies for Incorporating Exercise into Daily Life

Incorporating regular exercise into our daily lives is essential for maintaining good mental health and overall well-being. However, it can often be challenging to find the time and motivation to exercise consistently. This section will explore strategies that can help individuals incorporate exercise into their daily routines, making it a sustainable and enjoyable habit.

Setting Realistic and Attainable Goals

Setting realistic and attainable exercise goals is crucial when incorporating exercise into daily life. It is important to consider individual fitness levels, preferences, and time constraints. Setting goals that are too ambitious can lead to frustration and eventual discontinuation of the exercise routine.

To set realistic goals, individuals should consider factors such as their current fitness level, available time for exercise, and personal preferences. It is recommended to start with small, achievable goals and gradually increase the intensity and duration of the exercise as fitness levels improve. For example, setting a goal of 30 minutes of moderate-intensity exercise, three times a week, can be a realistic starting point for many individuals.

Finding Activities That Bring Joy

Incorporating exercise into daily life becomes easier when individuals find activities that bring them joy and satisfaction. Engaging in activities that are enjoyable increases motivation and makes exercise feel less like a chore.

The key is to explore different types of physical activities and find what resonates with personal preferences. Some individuals may enjoy outdoor activities such as hiking, biking, or swimming, while others may prefer group fitness classes or team sports. By finding an activity that brings joy, individuals are more likely to stick to their exercise routine and make it a regular part of their daily lives.

Scheduling Exercise as a Priority

Integrating exercise into daily life requires prioritizing it on the schedule. Just like any other important appointment or commitment, exercise deserves dedicated time.

One effective strategy is to schedule exercise at the same time every day or on specific days of the week. This creates a routine and helps individuals form the habit of regular exercise. For example, scheduling a morning workout before starting the day or planning evening walks after dinner can make exercise a priority.

Moreover, using calendars, reminder apps, or fitness trackers can serve as visual cues and help individuals stay accountable to their exercise schedule. By scheduling exercise as a priority, individuals are more likely to stay consistent and make exercise a regular part of their daily lives.

Incorporating Exercise into Daily Activities

Finding creative ways to incorporate exercise into daily activities can be a practical strategy for individuals with busy schedules. By making small adjustments to daily routines, individuals can increase overall physical activity levels without needing to find additional time for exercise.

Some simple strategies include taking the stairs instead of the elevator, parking the car a little farther away from the destination to include more walking, or incorporating short exercise breaks during work or study sessions. For example, doing a few minutes of stretching or light exercises every hour can help improve blood circulation and mental clarity.

Additionally, individuals can consider active modes of transportation, such as biking or walking, for short-distance trips instead of relying solely on motor vehicles. These small changes can accumulate over time and contribute to a more active lifestyle.

Accountability and Support

Accountability and support from others can significantly enhance the motivation to exercise regularly. Engaging in exercise with a partner, joining a fitness group or class, or hiring a personal trainer can provide the necessary support and accountability to stay committed to an exercise routine.

By having someone to exercise with or being part of a community, individuals can share their experiences, set goals together, and celebrate milestones. This not only creates a sense of belonging but also increases motivation and makes exercise more enjoyable.

Tracking Progress

Tracking progress can be a powerful strategy to stay motivated and committed to an exercise routine. This can be done through various methods, such as keeping an exercise journal, using fitness apps, or using wearable devices.

Tracking progress allows individuals to see their improvements over time, set new goals, and adjust their exercise routines accordingly. It provides a sense of achievement and helps maintain the momentum towards incorporating exercise into daily life.

Celebrating Achievements

Celebrating achievements, no matter how small, is essential to maintain motivation and create a positive association with exercise. By acknowledging and rewarding milestones, individuals reinforce the habit of exercising and are more likely to continue their efforts.

Celebrations can take various forms, such as treating oneself to a favorite healthy snack, purchasing new exercise gear, or enjoying a relaxing day off. These rewards not only provide a sense of accomplishment but also contribute to the overall well-being and satisfaction of incorporating exercise into daily life.

Conclusion

Incorporating exercise into daily life is crucial for maintaining good mental health and overall well-being. By setting realistic goals, finding activities that bring joy, scheduling exercise as a priority, incorporating exercise into daily activities, seeking accountability and support, tracking progress, and celebrating achievements, individuals can make exercise a sustainable and enjoyable part of their daily routines.

Developing a consistent exercise routine is a personal journey that requires patience and commitment. It is important to remember that everyone's journey is unique, and what works for one person may not work for another. Therefore, it is crucial to experiment with different strategies, adapt them to personal preferences, and find a routine that fits into individual lifestyles.

By incorporating exercise into daily life, individuals enhance their mental and physical well-being, improve overall quality of life, and pave the way for a healthier future. So, let's lace up those sneakers, find activities that bring joy, and embrace the transformative power of exercise.

Sleep and Mental Wellness

Importance of Sleep for Mental Health

Sleep plays a vital role in promoting mental health and overall well-being. It is a necessary physiological process that allows our bodies and minds to rest, recover, and rejuvenate. Adequate and quality sleep is essential for maintaining optimal brain function, emotional stability, and cognitive performance. In this section, we will explore the significance of sleep for mental health and discuss the potential consequences of sleep deprivation.

Sleep and Brain Function

Sleep is closely linked to various cognitive processes and neural functions. During sleep, the brain undergoes crucial restorative processes that are essential for memory consolidation, learning, and emotional regulation.

One of the key stages of sleep is known as REM (rapid eye movement) sleep, which is associated with vivid dreaming. REM sleep is crucial for emotional processing and regulation. It helps to consolidate emotional memories, process stressful experiences, and regulate mood. Lack of REM sleep has been linked to increased emotional reactivity, irritability, and mood disturbances.

Another important stage of sleep is NREM (non-rapid eye movement) sleep. NREM sleep is characterized by slower brain waves and is responsible for facilitating declarative memory consolidation, which is the ability to consciously recall facts and events. Insufficient NREM sleep can lead to difficulties in learning, attention, and problem-solving.

Additionally, sleep is essential for maintaining proper cognitive function, such as attention, concentration, and decision-making. Sleep deprivation has been shown to impair cognitive performance, including decreased attention span, reduced working memory capacity, and slower reaction times.

Sleep and Mental Wellness

The relationship between sleep and mental health is bidirectional. On one hand, mental health conditions, such as anxiety disorders, depression, and bipolar disorder, can disrupt normal sleep patterns. On the other hand, chronic sleep deprivation or poor sleep quality can increase the risk of developing mental health problems.

Anxiety disorders and sleep disorders often coexist and can exacerbate one another. Sleep disturbances, such as insomnia or nightmares, are common symptoms of anxiety disorders. Conversely, chronic sleep deprivation or disrupted sleep can increase anxiety levels and contribute to the development or worsening of anxiety disorders.

Depression is strongly linked to sleep disturbances. Insomnia is a prevalent symptom of depression, and individuals with insomnia have a higher risk of developing depression. Sleep deprivation disrupts the balance of chemicals in the brain that regulate mood, such as serotonin and dopamine, which can contribute to the development of depressive symptoms.

Bipolar disorder is characterized by extreme mood swings, and disruptions in sleep patterns are a hallmark of this condition. Both manic and depressive episodes can lead to changes in sleep duration and quality. Sleep disturbances can trigger or exacerbate bipolar symptoms, and managing sleep patterns is an important aspect of bipolar disorder treatment.

Consequences of Sleep Deprivation

Insufficient sleep and chronic sleep deprivation can have significant negative consequences for mental health and well-being. Prolonged sleep deprivation disrupts the brain's ability to function optimally, leading to a range of physical, emotional, and cognitive problems.

The immediate effects of sleep deprivation include decreased alertness, impaired concentration, and memory problems. These effects can impact daily activities, productivity, and job performance. Lack of sleep can also compromise decision-making abilities and increase the risk of accidents, both at home and in the workplace.

In the long term, chronic sleep deprivation is associated with an increased risk of developing mental health disorders. Sleep deprivation can contribute to the development of mood disorders, such as depression and anxiety. It can also worsen existing mental health conditions and increase the severity of symptoms.

Sleep deprivation has been linked to a higher risk of developing psychotic disorders, such as schizophrenia. Disruptions in the sleep-wake cycle and abnormal sleep patterns are common features of schizophrenia, and sleep disturbances can influence the onset and progression of the illness.

Furthermore, chronic sleep deprivation weakens the immune system and increases susceptibility to infections and illnesses. It can also contribute to the development of chronic health conditions, such as cardiovascular diseases, obesity, and diabetes, which can further impact mental health.

Strategies for Improving Sleep Quality

Given the critical role of sleep in mental health, it is important to prioritize good sleep hygiene and adopt strategies that promote quality sleep. Here are some tips to improve sleep quality:

1. Establish a regular sleep schedule: Going to bed and waking up at consistent times helps regulate the body's internal clock and promotes healthy sleep patterns.

2. Create a sleep-friendly environment: Ensure that your bedroom is quiet, dark, and at a comfortable temperature. Use earplugs, eye masks, or white noise machines if necessary.

3. Practice a relaxing bedtime routine: Engage in calming activities before bed, such as reading a book, taking a warm bath, or practicing relaxation techniques like deep breathing or meditation.

4. Limit exposure to screens before bed: The blue light emitted by electronic devices can interfere with sleep. Avoid using screens for at least an hour before bedtime.

5. Avoid stimulating substances: Limit caffeine and nicotine intake, especially in the evening, as they can disrupt sleep. Alcohol may initially induce sleep but can lead to poor sleep quality later in the night.

6. Exercise regularly: Engaging in physical activity during the day can promote better sleep at night. However, avoid intense exercise close to bedtime, as it can interfere with falling asleep.

7. Manage stress: High levels of stress can make it difficult to fall asleep or stay asleep. Practice stress management techniques, such as mindfulness, journaling, or seeking support from a therapist.

8. Seek professional help if needed: If you are experiencing chronic sleep problems or suspect an underlying sleep disorder, consult a healthcare professional for a comprehensive evaluation and appropriate treatment.

Remember, ensuring adequate and restful sleep is an important aspect of maintaining good mental health. By prioritizing sleep and adopting healthy sleep habits, you can significantly contribute to your overall well-being.

Common Sleep Disorders and Their Effects on Mental Health

Sleep is a fundamental aspect of overall health and well-being. It plays a crucial role in physical restoration, cognitive functioning, mood regulation, and emotional well-being. However, many individuals experience difficulties with sleep, which can significantly impact their mental health. In this section, we will explore some common sleep disorders and their effects on mental health.

Insomnia

Insomnia is the most prevalent sleep disorder, affecting approximately one-third of the population at some point in their lives. It is characterized by difficulty falling asleep, staying asleep, or experiencing non-restorative sleep. Chronic insomnia, which lasts for at least three months, can have profound effects on mental health.

Individuals with insomnia are at an increased risk of developing mood disorders, such as depression and anxiety. Persistent sleep deprivation can lead to an imbalance in neurotransmitters, such as serotonin and dopamine, which play a crucial role in regulating mood and emotions. Moreover, the chronic activation of the stress response system due to insomnia can contribute to the development of anxiety disorders.

Example: Sarah, a 35-year-old woman, has been struggling with chronic insomnia for several years. She often lies awake at night, unable to fall asleep despite feeling exhausted. As a result, she feels constantly fatigued, irritable, and has difficulty concentrating during the day. Sarah's insomnia has taken a toll on her mental health, leading to symptoms of depression and anxiety.

Sleep Apnea

Sleep apnea is a sleep disorder characterized by pauses in breathing or shallow breaths during sleep. It is often accompanied by snoring and repeated awakenings throughout the night. Sleep apnea can have significant consequences for mental health.

The fragmented and poor-quality sleep associated with sleep apnea can lead to daytime sleepiness, fatigue, and cognitive impairments. These factors can contribute to the development or worsening of mood disorders, such as depression and irritability. Additionally, sleep apnea has been linked to an increased risk of cardiovascular problems, which can further impact mental health.

Example: John, a 50-year-old man, has been diagnosed with moderate obstructive sleep apnea. He frequently wakes up throughout the night gasping for breath and experiences excessive daytime sleepiness. John's sleep apnea has not only affected his physical health but has also contributed to his feelings of irritability and low mood.

Restless Legs Syndrome (RLS)

Restless Legs Syndrome (RLS) is a neurological disorder characterized by an uncontrollable urge to move the legs, often accompanied by uncomfortable sensations. These sensations typically occur or worsen during periods of rest or inactivity, such as when trying to fall asleep. RLS can significantly disrupt sleep, leading to various mental health challenges.

The sleep disturbances caused by RLS can result in chronic sleep deprivation and daytime fatigue. The lack of quality sleep can contribute to the development of mood disorders, including depression and anxiety. Furthermore, the discomfort and restlessness experienced during bedtime can lead to heightened levels of stress and frustration, negatively impacting overall mental well-being.

Example: Emily, a 40-year-old woman, has been dealing with symptoms of Restless Legs Syndrome (RLS) for the past few years. She experiences an irresistible urge to move her legs, particularly when she lies down to sleep. As a result, she struggles to fall asleep and often feels exhausted and moody during the day. Emily's RLS has significantly affected her mental health, leading to increased feelings of frustration and distress.

Sleep-Wake Schedule Disorders

Sleep-wake schedule disorders refer to disruptions in the timing of sleep and wakefulness. Common examples include delayed sleep phase disorder (DSPD) and shift work disorder. These disorders can have significant implications for mental health.

Individuals with sleep-wake schedule disorders often struggle with maintaining consistent sleep patterns. This can result in chronic sleep deprivation, leading to difficulties with mood regulation, concentration, and overall cognitive functioning. The misalignment between their internal biological clock and the social demands of their daily life can contribute to increased levels of stress, anxiety, and even symptoms resembling depression.

Example: Mark, a 28-year-old man, works night shifts as a nurse, which has disrupted his sleep-wake schedule. He struggles to fall asleep during the day and often feels fatigued and irritable when awake. Mark's irregular sleep schedule has had a significant impact on his mental health, contributing to feelings of anxiety and low mood.

Narcolepsy

Narcolepsy is a neurological disorder characterized by excessive daytime sleepiness, sudden loss of muscle tone (cataplexy), and vivid hallucinations while falling asleep or waking up. People with narcolepsy often struggle with maintaining regular sleep-wake cycles, which can have profound effects on mental health.

The excessive daytime sleepiness experienced by individuals with narcolepsy can lead to difficulties in functioning throughout the day. This can result in impaired cognitive performance, decreased motivation, and feelings of frustration or irritability. Moreover, the unpredictable nature of narcoleptic symptoms can cause stress and anxiety, further impacting mental well-being.

Example: Alex, a 22-year-old college student, has been diagnosed with narcolepsy. He frequently experiences episodes of excessive daytime sleepiness, even after getting a full night's rest. Alex's narcolepsy has made it challenging for him to concentrate in class, leading to feelings of frustration and low self-esteem.

In conclusion, sleep disorders can have significant impacts on mental health. Insomnia, sleep apnea, restless legs syndrome, sleep-wake schedule disorders, and narcolepsy all disrupt the sleep-wake cycle, leading to various mental health challenges. It is essential to recognize and address these sleep disorders in order to promote overall well-being and support individuals in achieving optimal mental health.

Strategies for Improving Sleep Quality

Getting good quality sleep is essential for maintaining mental health and overall well-being. However, many people struggle with sleep-related issues, which can have a significant impact on their daily functioning and quality of life. In this section, we will explore various strategies that can help improve sleep quality and promote better mental health.

Establishing a Consistent Sleep Routine

One of the most effective strategies for improving sleep quality is establishing a consistent sleep routine. Our bodies have a natural internal clock, known as the circadian rhythm, which regulates our sleep-wake cycle. By going to bed and waking up at the same time every day, we can synchronize our internal clock and promote better sleep. Consistency in sleep routine helps regulate our body's melatonin production, a hormone that plays a crucial role in promoting sleep.

To establish a consistent sleep routine, it is important to prioritize sleep and set aside enough time for it. Create a relaxing bedtime routine that signals to your body that it is time to wind down and prepare for sleep. This could include activities such as reading a book, taking a warm bath, or practicing relaxation techniques like deep breathing or meditation.

Creating a Sleep-Friendly Environment

Creating a sleep-friendly environment plays a vital role in improving sleep quality. Your sleep environment should be quiet, dark, and cool. Ensure that your bedroom is free from distractions and that your bed and pillows are comfortable and supportive. Consider investing in blackout curtains, earplugs, or a white noise machine if you live in a noisy area.

It is also important to limit your exposure to electronics, especially blue light emitted by electronic devices like smartphones, tablets, and computers. Blue light can suppress the production of melatonin and disrupt your sleep. Avoid using electronics at least an hour before bedtime, or use blue light filters or amber-toned glasses to reduce your exposure.

Managing Stress and Anxiety

Stress and anxiety can significantly impact sleep quality. It is essential to develop effective stress management strategies to promote better sleep. Engaging in relaxation techniques, such as deep breathing exercises, progressive muscle relaxation, or guided imagery, can help calm an overactive mind and prepare the body for sleep.

Practicing mindfulness meditation can also be beneficial in reducing stress and promoting better sleep. Mindfulness involves paying attention to the present moment, without judgment. Regular practice of mindfulness meditation has been shown to improve sleep quality and reduce symptoms of insomnia.

Adopting Healthy Lifestyle Habits

Certain lifestyle habits can have a significant impact on sleep quality. Here are some key strategies to promote better sleep:

- Regular exercise: Engaging in regular physical activity can help improve sleep quality. However, it is important to time your exercise appropriately. Avoid intense exercise close to bedtime, as it can increase alertness and make it difficult to fall asleep.

- Limit caffeine and alcohol intake: Caffeine is a stimulant that can interfere with sleep. Limit your consumption of caffeinated beverages like coffee, tea, and energy drinks, especially in the afternoon and evening. Although alcohol can make you feel drowsy initially, it can disrupt your sleep later in the night.

- Avoid large meals and heavy snacks before bedtime: Eating heavy or spicy meals before bedtime can cause discomfort and make it harder to fall asleep. It is best to have a light snack if needed.

- Create a calm and relaxing bedtime routine: Engaging in activities that promote relaxation before bedtime can help prepare your body for sleep. This can include reading a book, taking a warm bath, or practicing relaxation exercises.

- Avoid napping late in the day: While short power naps can be beneficial, taking long naps or napping late in the day can interfere with nighttime sleep. If you need to nap, keep it brief (around 20-30 minutes) and avoid napping after 3 pm.

- Maintain a comfortable sleep environment: Ensure that your bedroom is cool, quiet, and comfortable. Use comfortable pillows and a supportive mattress that suits your personal preferences.

- Limit exposure to stimulating activities before bed: Engaging in stimulating activities before bedtime, such as working on a computer or watching intense movies, can make it harder to fall asleep. Create a relaxing routine that helps transition your mind and body into a sleep-ready state.

Seeking Professional Help

If you have tried various strategies to improve sleep quality and still struggle with sleep issues, it may be beneficial to seek professional help. A healthcare provider or a sleep specialist can evaluate your sleep patterns, identify any underlying sleep disorders, and recommend appropriate interventions or treatments.

There are various treatment options available for sleep disorders, including medications, cognitive-behavioral therapy for insomnia (CBT-I), and other specialized therapies. Seeking professional help can provide you with personalized guidance and support to improve your sleep quality and overall well-being.

Summary

Improving sleep quality is crucial for maintaining good mental health and overall well-being. By establishing a consistent sleep routine, creating a sleep-friendly environment, managing stress and anxiety, adopting healthy lifestyle habits, and seeking professional help when needed, you can work towards achieving better sleep and improved mental wellness.

Remember that everyone's sleep needs and preferences are different, so it might take some trial and error to find the strategies that work best for you. Be patient and persistent in your efforts to improve sleep quality, knowing that the benefits will extend to all areas of your life.

Social Support and Connection

The Significance of Social Support in Mental Health

Social support plays a vital role in mental health and wellbeing. It encompasses various aspects of interpersonal relationships, including emotional, informational, and practical support from individuals, communities, and social networks. In this section, we will explore the significance of social support in promoting mental health, the positive effects it has on individuals, and strategies for fostering and maintaining supportive relationships.

Understanding Social Support

To understand the significance of social support in mental health, we need to first grasp its different dimensions. Social support can be categorized into four main types:

1. Emotional support: This type of support involves the expression of empathy, love, trust, and care. It provides individuals with a sense of belonging and security. Examples of emotional support include listening, offering encouragement, and providing reassurance during challenging times.

2. Informational support: This support relates to the provision of advice, guidance, and information. It helps individuals gain knowledge, solve problems, and make informed decisions. Examples of informational support include educating someone about available mental health resources or providing guidance on accessing treatment options.

3. Instrumental support: Instrumental support is tangible assistance in the form of practical help or resources. It addresses the individual's concrete needs and aids

in meeting daily requirements. Examples of instrumental support include financial assistance, help with daily chores, or transportation to appointments.

4. Appraisal support: This type of support involves the provision of feedback, evaluation, and affirmation. It helps individuals gain a new perspective on their situations and enhance their coping abilities. Examples of appraisal support include constructive feedback, validation of feelings, and helping someone reframe their thoughts.

The Positive Effects of Social Support

Numerous studies have shown that social support has positive effects on mental health and wellbeing. Some of the key benefits of social support include:

1. Buffering against stress: Social support acts as a buffer against the negative impact of stress on mental health. It provides individuals with a sense of security, reduces feelings of isolation, and helps them cope with challenging situations.

2. Increased resilience: Having a strong support system fosters resilience, enabling individuals to bounce back from adversity and adapt to changes effectively. Social support provides emotional resources and coping strategies to navigate through difficult times.

3. Enhanced self-esteem: Positive relationships and supportive networks contribute to a sense of belonging, acceptance, and validation. This, in turn, bolsters self-esteem and self-worth, positively influencing mental wellbeing.

4. Improved treatment outcomes: Social support plays a crucial role in treatment adherence and recovery. Having supportive individuals around can encourage engagement in therapy, medication compliance, and overall treatment participation.

5. Reduced risk of mental health disorders: Strong social support networks have been linked to a lower risk of developing mental health disorders such as depression, anxiety, and substance abuse. Social connection and meaningful relationships act as protective factors.

Strategies for Building and Maintaining Supportive Relationships

Building and maintaining supportive relationships require effort and intentionality. Here are some strategies to foster social support:

1. Cultivate quality relationships: Focus on developing deep, meaningful connections with a few individuals rather than having a large number of superficial relationships. Invest time and energy into nurturing these relationships.

2. Seek out support: Actively reach out to others when you are in need. Don't hesitate to ask for help or express your emotions. People often appreciate the opportunity to provide support and feel valued when they are trusted.

3. Join support groups: Consider joining support groups or community organizations that align with your interests or experiences. These groups provide an opportunity to connect with others who have similar backgrounds or challenges.

4. Build reciprocal relationships: Social support should be a two-way street. Be there for others when they need support, and they will be more likely to reciprocate. Healthy relationships involve mutual care and investment.

5. Utilize technology for connection: In our digital age, technology offers various avenues for social connection. Engage in online communities, support forums, or virtual mental health support groups to find like-minded individuals and receive support.

6. Foster a sense of belonging: Create inclusive environments where everyone feels valued and heard. Encourage open communication, empathy, and respect in your social circles, workplaces, or communities.

7. Practice active listening: Enhance your communication skills by actively listening to others. Show genuine interest, empathy, and understanding. Validating someone's experiences can make them feel supported and cherished.

Remember that social support is a dynamic process that requires ongoing effort. It is essential to cultivate and maintain supportive relationships as part of a holistic approach to mental health and overall wellbeing.

Real-World Example: The Role of Support Groups

Support groups are a prime example of social support in action. These groups bring together individuals facing similar challenges, providing them with a space to share experiences, exchange information, and offer emotional support. Let's consider the example of a support group for individuals with anxiety disorders:

Sarah has been struggling with severe anxiety for several years. Despite therapy and medication, she often feels isolated and misunderstood. She decides to join a local anxiety support group, where she meets people who share similar struggles. Through the group, Sarah finds a supportive community that understands her experiences, offers coping strategies, and listens without judgment. The support group becomes a valuable source of social support for Sarah, boosting her mental wellbeing and providing her with a sense of belonging.

Additional Resources

1. *Lost Connections: Uncovering the Real Causes of Depression – and the Unexpected Solutions* by Johann Hari. This book explores the importance of social connections and challenges the prevailing biomedical model of mental health.

2. National Alliance on Mental Illness (NAMI) Helpline: 1-800-950-NAMI (6264) NAMI provides support, education, and advocacy for individuals and families affected by mental health conditions. Their helpline offers information and resources for seeking help and support.

Key Takeaways

1. Social support, encompassing emotional, informational, instrumental, and appraisal support, plays a significant role in mental health and wellbeing.

2. Social support acts as a buffer against stress, enhances resilience, improves self-esteem, and positively influences treatment outcomes.

3. Strategies for building and maintaining supportive relationships include cultivating quality connections, seeking support, joining support groups, utilizing technology, and practicing active listening.

4. Support groups are real-world examples of social support in action, providing individuals with a sense of community and understanding.

Remember that social support is not a one-size-fits-all approach. Each person's needs and preferences may differ, so individuals should explore and find the types and sources of social support that work best for them. By fostering and maintaining social support networks, individuals can enhance their mental health and overall wellbeing.

So, let's recognize the significance of social support in promoting mental health and strive to cultivate meaningful connections in our lives.

Building and Maintaining Supportive Relationships

Building and maintaining supportive relationships is a critical aspect of mental health and overall wellbeing. Human beings are social creatures by nature, and having healthy connections with others has been shown to have numerous benefits for mental wellness. In this section, we will explore the importance of social support, strategies for fostering supportive relationships, and the role of community and social networks in promoting mental wellbeing.

The Significance of Social Support in Mental Health

Social support refers to the assistance, care, and validation that individuals receive from their social connections, including family, friends, colleagues, and community members. It plays a vital role in mental health by providing emotional support, instrumental support, and informational support.

Emotional support involves providing comfort, empathy, and understanding during challenging times. It helps individuals feel valued and nurtured, reducing feelings of loneliness and isolation. Instrumental support refers to the tangible assistance that others provide, such as helping with practical tasks or providing financial support. Lastly, informational support involves sharing knowledge, advice, and guidance, providing individuals with valuable insights and resources.

Research has consistently shown that social support is associated with better mental health outcomes. Individuals with strong social support networks experience lower levels of stress, anxiety, and depression. They also have higher self-esteem and a greater sense of life satisfaction. Conversely, lack of social support has been linked to increased risk of mental health disorders and poorer overall wellbeing.

Building and Maintaining Supportive Relationships

Developing and nurturing supportive relationships requires effort and intentionality. Here are some strategies to help build and maintain these connections:

1. Foster open communication: Open and honest communication is the foundation of any healthy relationship. Expressing emotions, thoughts, and needs in a respectful manner fosters understanding and creates a safe space for vulnerability.

2. Cultivate empathy and active listening: Empathy involves putting yourself in someone else's shoes and seeking to understand their experiences and perspectives. Active listening, on the other hand, involves fully engaging with the person speaking

and giving them your full attention. Both empathy and active listening promote deeper connections and a sense of validation.

3. Show appreciation and gratitude: Expressing appreciation and gratitude towards others strengthens the bond between individuals. Acknowledge and thank your loved ones for their support and let them know that you value their presence in your life.

4. Offer support and be reliable: Being there for others in times of need is crucial for building supportive relationships. Offer a helping hand, lend a listening ear, and be dependable. Consistency and reliability build trust and reinforce the idea that the relationship is a safe space for sharing struggles and joys.

5. Respect boundaries: Respecting personal boundaries is crucial for maintaining healthy relationships. Understand and honor each other's limits and preferences. Recognize that everyone has different needs for solitude or personal space.

6. Engage in shared activities: Engaging in shared activities and hobbies helps strengthen bonds and create new opportunities for connection. Find activities that you enjoy together and make time to engage in them regularly.

7. Seek professional help when needed: Sometimes, building and maintaining supportive relationships can be challenging, especially when facing complex personal issues or mental health disorders. Seeking the help of a therapist or counselor can provide guidance and support in navigating these difficulties.

The Role of Community and Social Networks in Mental Wellbeing

Supportive relationships extend beyond individual connections and can involve larger communities and social networks. The sense of belonging and social integration that comes from being part of a community has significant benefits for mental wellbeing. Here are some ways in which communities and social networks contribute to mental health:

1. Sense of belonging: Being part of a community provides individuals with a sense of belonging and purpose. It helps combat feelings of isolation and loneliness that can negatively impact mental health.

2. Social engagement: Community involvement promotes social engagement, which has been shown to have numerous mental health benefits. Participating in group activities, volunteering, or joining clubs and organizations can foster new connections and enhance social support.

3. Norms and values: Communities often have shared norms, values, and beliefs that can positively influence individuals' mental health. These values can promote

inclusivity, diversity, and acceptance, creating an environment where individuals can feel understood and supported.

4. Resources and support services: Communities often offer various resources and support services to promote mental wellbeing. These can include mental health clinics, support groups, helplines, and community-based initiatives focused on mental health awareness and advocacy.

5. Reducing stigma: Communities have the power to challenge and reduce the stigma surrounding mental health. By fostering open conversations and promoting education, communities can create an environment where individuals feel comfortable seeking help and support.

Conclusion

Building and maintaining supportive relationships is essential for mental health and overall wellbeing. The presence of social support contributes to lower levels of stress, improved self-esteem, and greater life satisfaction. By fostering open communication, cultivating empathy, showing appreciation, and respecting boundaries, individuals can create and nurture strong connections.

Additionally, being part of a community and engaging with social networks can provide a sense of belonging, access to resources, and opportunities for social engagement. Communities play a crucial role in reducing stigma and promoting mental health awareness.

As we continue to explore transformative approaches to mental health and wellbeing, it is important to recognize and prioritize the role of supportive relationships in shaping the future of wellness. By prioritizing and investing in these connections, we can create a mental health landscape that fosters resilience, growth, and collective wellbeing.

The Role of Community and Social Networks in Mental Wellbeing

Community and social networks play a vital role in promoting and maintaining mental wellbeing. In this section, we will explore the importance of social support, the impact of relationships on mental health, and strategies for building and nurturing supportive networks.

The Importance of Social Support

Social support refers to the assistance, comfort, and validation that individuals receive from their social relationships. It encompasses emotional, informational, and instrumental support, all of which contribute to an individual's overall wellbeing.

Research consistently shows that social support is a significant protective factor against mental health problems. People who have strong social connections and support systems tend to experience lower levels of stress, depression, and anxiety. On the other hand, individuals with limited social support are at a higher risk of developing mental health issues.

The Impact of Relationships on Mental Health

The quality and nature of relationships have a profound impact on mental health. Positive, healthy relationships can provide a sense of belonging, acceptance, and love, which are crucial for emotional well-being. Conversely, toxic or unhealthy relationships can cause distress, negatively impact self-esteem, and contribute to mental health problems.

Close, intimate relationships, such as those with romantic partners or best friends, have been found to be particularly influential in promoting mental wellbeing. These relationships provide emotional support, companionship, and a safe space for self-disclosure and vulnerability. They can help buffer against the negative effects of stress and provide a sense of security and stability.

Beyond intimate relationships, broader social networks also play a role in mental wellbeing. Having a diverse network of friends, acquaintances, and colleagues can provide a sense of social integration and connectedness. These connections offer opportunities for socializing, engaging in meaningful activities, and receiving different forms of support.

Building and Maintaining Supportive Relationships

Developing and maintaining supportive relationships is essential for mental wellbeing. Here are some strategies to consider:

1. Cultivate meaningful connections: Seek out relationships that are based on mutual trust, respect, and shared values. Invest time and effort in building deep connections with others.

2. Communicate openly: Effective communication is key in maintaining healthy relationships. Practice active listening, empathy, and assertiveness to enhance understanding and resolve conflicts constructively.

3. Offer and seek support: Be willing to provide support to others when they are in need. Similarly, don't hesitate to reach out and ask for help when you require it.

4. Foster a sense of belonging: Engage in activities and communities that align with your interests and values. Participating in shared experiences can help foster a sense of belonging and facilitate the formation of new relationships.

5. Embrace diversity: Connect with people from different backgrounds and with varied perspectives. Embracing diversity can broaden your social network and enrich your understanding of the world.

6. Utilize technology wisely: While technology can facilitate social connections, it's important to strike a healthy balance. Ensure that online interactions supplement, rather than substitute, face-to-face interactions.

The Role of Community and Social Networks in Mental Wellbeing

Community and social networks act as a supportive framework that contributes to mental wellbeing in several ways:

1. Providing emotional support: Communities offer a sense of belonging and validation that can help individuals cope with stress, trauma, and other mental health challenges. Supportive communities create safe spaces for individuals to share their experiences and receive empathy and understanding.

2. Building resilience: Social networks can enhance an individual's ability to bounce back from adversity. Through support and encouragement, communities can facilitate the development of resilience and coping skills, which are essential in maintaining mental wellbeing.

3. Offering resources and information: Communities often provide access to resources and information related to mental health services, support groups, and educational programs. These resources can empower individuals to seek appropriate help and make informed decisions about their mental health.

4. Reducing stigma and discrimination: Communities have the power to challenge and reduce the stigma and discrimination surrounding mental health. By fostering understanding and acceptance, communities can create an environment that supports individuals with mental health concerns and encourages seeking help.

5. Promoting social inclusion: Social networks and communities promote social inclusion by providing opportunities for individuals to participate in group activities, collaborate on projects, and engage with others. This sense of inclusion can enhance self-esteem and overall mental wellbeing.

In conclusion, community and social networks play a crucial role in promoting mental wellbeing. It is important to recognize the significance of social support in maintaining mental health and take proactive steps to build and nurture supportive relationships and communities. By doing so, we can create a more compassionate and resilient society that values and prioritizes mental wellbeing.

Self-Care Practices

Understanding Self-Care and Its Importance for Mental Wellness

Self-care is a critical aspect of maintaining and enhancing mental wellness. It involves taking deliberate actions to prioritize one's physical, emotional, and psychological well-being. By engaging in self-care practices, individuals can nurture themselves and prevent or alleviate mental health challenges.

The Concept of Self-Care

Self-care encompasses a wide range of activities that promote self-nourishment and support overall mental wellness. It involves recognizing one's needs and actively taking steps to fulfill them. Self-care is not selfish; rather, it is an essential practice that allows individuals to recharge, manage stress, and maintain a healthy balance in their lives.

Self-care practices can vary from person to person, as they are highly individualized. Some common self-care activities include engaging in hobbies, practicing relaxation techniques, engaging in physical activity, spending time in nature, maintaining social connections, seeking therapy, and practicing mindfulness. It is important to note that self-care is not limited to any specific activity, but rather, it is a mindset that prioritizes one's well-being.

The Importance of Self-Care

Self-care plays a vital role in promoting and maintaining mental wellness. It is an essential aspect of preventing burnout, managing stress, and building resilience. Here are some key reasons why self-care is crucial for mental well-being:

- **Stress Reduction:** Engaging in self-care activities helps to reduce stress levels. When individuals prioritize their well-being, they can better cope with daily stressors and prevent the accumulation of stress over time. Self-care techniques, such as deep breathing exercises, meditation, or taking breaks, can help individuals relax and rejuvenate.

- **Improved Emotional Well-being:** Self-care contributes to emotional well-being by allowing individuals to tune in to their emotions and address them effectively. Engaging in activities that bring joy, such as pursuing hobbies or spending time with loved ones, can boost mood and help manage emotions in a healthy way.

- **Enhanced Physical Health:** Taking care of one's physical health is an integral part of self-care. Engaging in regular exercise, eating a balanced diet, and getting enough sleep not only benefit physical health but also have a positive impact on mental well-being. Physical well-being and mental well-being are closely interconnected.

- **Building Resilience:** Self-care practices build resilience by strengthening individuals' ability to cope with challenges and setbacks. By prioritizing their well-being, individuals develop the tools and strategies necessary to overcome adversity and maintain mental wellness. Self-care helps individuals bounce back from stress and maintain a positive outlook.

- **Preventing Burnout:** Engaging in self-care helps prevent burnout, which is often caused by chronic stress and overexertion. Burnout can lead to emotional exhaustion, reduced productivity, and a decreased sense of fulfillment. Regular self-care activities provide individuals with the necessary downtime to recharge and prevent burnout.

Strategies for Practicing Self-Care

Developing a personalized self-care routine is essential for maintaining mental wellness. Here are some strategies to help individuals integrate self-care into their daily lives:

- **Identify Personal Needs:** Start by identifying your personal needs and what activities or practices promote your well-being. Reflect on what brings you joy, reduces stress, and helps you feel rejuvenated. These activities will form the foundation of your self-care routine.

- **Create a Self-Care Plan:** Develop a self-care plan that encompasses your identified needs and activities. Schedule regular time for self-care and make it a non-negotiable part of your routine. Incorporate a variety of activities that cater to different aspects of your well-being, such as physical, emotional, and social needs.

- **Practice Mindfulness:** Cultivate mindfulness by being fully present in the moment and paying attention to your thoughts, emotions, and sensations.

This can be done through mindful breathing exercises, meditation, or simply taking a few moments each day to pause and observe your surroundings without judgment.

- **Set Boundaries:** Establish clear boundaries to protect your time and energy. Learn to say no to commitments or activities that do not align with your self-care priorities. Boundaries ensure that you have the necessary time and space to take care of yourself.

- **Engage in Activities That Bring Joy:** Make time for activities that bring you joy and allow you to relax and unwind. Whether it's reading a book, pursuing a hobby, or spending time in nature, engaging in activities that bring joy helps boost mood and overall well-being.

- **Seek Support:** Reach out to loved ones, friends, or professionals for support when needed. Building a support system and fostering meaningful connections is an essential part of self-care. Share your thoughts, emotions, and challenges with trusted individuals who can provide a listening ear and offer guidance.

Challenges and Barriers to Self-Care

While self-care is essential, there can be challenges and barriers that hinder individuals from prioritizing their well-being. Here are some common challenges and strategies to overcome them:

- **Limited Time:** Busy schedules and competing responsibilities can make it challenging to find time for self-care. However, even small pockets of time can be utilized for self-care. Prioritize activities that bring you joy and make self-care a non-negotiable part of your routine.

- **Guilt or Self-Criticism:** Some individuals may feel guilty or self-critical for prioritizing their own needs. It is important to recognize that self-care is not selfish, but rather, it is necessary for overall well-being. Challenge any negative self-talk and practice self-compassion.

- **Lack of Knowledge:** Some individuals may be unaware of the importance of self-care or the various practices they can engage in. Educate yourself about self-care and explore different strategies to find what works best for you. Experiment with different activities and techniques to discover what brings you joy and relaxation.

- **Financial Constraints:** Certain self-care activities may require financial resources, such as attending a yoga class or getting a massage. However, self-care does not have to be costly. Many activities, such as taking a walk in nature or practicing deep breathing exercises, are accessible and free. Focus on activities that align with your budget.

In conclusion, self-care is a fundamental aspect of mental wellness. By prioritizing and engaging in self-care practices, individuals can enhance their emotional well-being, reduce stress, build resilience, and prevent burnout. It is essential to develop a personalized self-care routine and overcome challenges or barriers that may hinder self-care. Remember, self-care is not a luxury but a necessity for maintaining and enhancing mental wellness.

Strategies for Developing a Personalized Self-Care Routine

Developing a personalized self-care routine is crucial for maintaining and promoting mental wellness. Self-care involves intentionally taking care of oneself, both physically and emotionally, to ensure overall well-being. In this section, we will explore various strategies and techniques that individuals can incorporate into their lives to create a personalized self-care routine.

Identify and Prioritize Your Needs

The first step in developing a personalized self-care routine is to identify and prioritize your needs. Take some time to reflect on what aspects of your life contribute to your overall well-being. Consider your physical, emotional, and social needs. Ask yourself the following questions:

- What activities bring me joy and relaxation?

- What are my stress triggers, and how can I minimize their impact?

- Which relationships in my life nurture and support me?

- How do I recharge and rejuvenate?

By answering these questions, you can gain insight into areas where you need to focus your self-care efforts.

Create a Self-Care Plan

Once you have identified your needs, it's time to create a self-care plan. A self-care plan outlines the activities and strategies you will incorporate into your routine to meet your needs. Here are some steps to help you create an effective plan:

1. Set realistic goals: Start by setting specific, achievable goals for your self-care routine. For example, you might aim to dedicate 30 minutes each day to engage in activities that promote relaxation.

2. Choose self-care activities: Select activities that align with your identified needs and goals. These activities can be as simple as taking a walk in nature, practicing mindfulness, or engaging in a hobby you enjoy. Remember, self-care is highly personal, so choose activities that resonate with you.

3. Plan for consistency: Consistency is key when it comes to self-care. Schedule regular time slots for your self-care activities, and treat them as non-negotiable appointments with yourself. Consider integrating self-care practices into your daily or weekly routine for maximum impact.

4. Be flexible: While consistency is important, it's also essential to be flexible and open to adjusting your self-care plan as needed. Life can be unpredictable, and circumstances may change. Adapt your routine accordingly, and don't be too hard on yourself if things don't go as planned.

Practice Self-Compassion

Self-compassion is a fundamental aspect of self-care. It involves treating yourself with kindness, understanding, and acceptance, especially during challenging times. Here are some strategies to cultivate self-compassion:

- Practice positive self-talk: Replace self-critical thoughts with compassionate and encouraging self-talk. Remind yourself that it's okay to prioritize your own well-being.

- Set realistic expectations: Avoid setting unrealistic expectations for yourself. Recognize your limits and embrace imperfections.

- Celebrate small victories: Acknowledge and celebrate your achievements, no matter how small they may seem. Reward yourself for your efforts, and give yourself credit for your progress.

Engage in Self-Care Activities

Now that you have a self-care plan in place, it's time to engage in self-care activities. Here are some examples of self-care practices you can include in your routine:

- Physical self-care: Engage in regular exercise, prioritize sleep, practice good nutrition, and take care of your physical health.
- Emotional self-care: Journaling, practicing gratitude, engaging in creative activities, and seeking support from loved ones are all examples of emotional self-care.
- Social self-care: Foster and maintain healthy relationships, spend quality time with loved ones, join social groups or clubs, and engage in meaningful conversations.
- Mental self-care: Engage in activities that challenge and stimulate your mind, such as reading, puzzles, or learning new skills.

Evaluate and Adjust

Regularly evaluate the effectiveness of your self-care routine and make adjustments as needed. Check-in with yourself to determine if the activities you've chosen are truly meeting your needs. Be open to trying new strategies and techniques, and don't be afraid to ask for help or seek guidance from professionals if necessary.

Remember, self-care is an ongoing process, and it may take time to find what truly works for you. Be patient and persistent, as developing a personalized self-care routine is a powerful tool for promoting mental well-being.

Conclusion

In this section, we explored strategies for developing a personalized self-care routine. By identifying and prioritizing your needs, creating a self-care plan, practicing self-compassion, engaging in self-care activities, and regularly evaluating and adjusting your routine, you can cultivate a strong foundation for mental well-being. Self-care is a lifelong journey, and by dedicating time and attention to your own needs, you can navigate life's challenges with resilience and positivity.

Challenges and Barriers to Self-Care

Self-care is an essential aspect of maintaining mental wellness. It refers to the deliberate actions individuals take to care for their own physical, emotional, and mental well-being. While self-care can have numerous benefits, including stress reduction, improved mood, and increased resilience, there are also challenges and barriers that individuals may face in implementing self-care practices. In this section, we will explore some of these challenges and barriers and discuss strategies to overcome them.

Time Constraints

One of the most common challenges to self-care is the perception of not having enough time. Many individuals, especially those juggling multiple responsibilities such as work, family, and personal commitments, may find it difficult to prioritize self-care activities. The demands of everyday life can make it challenging to carve out dedicated time for self-care practices.

To overcome this barrier, it is important to recognize that self-care does not have to be time-consuming. It can involve small activities that can be easily integrated into daily routines. For example, taking short breaks during the day to practice deep breathing exercises, going for a walk during lunch breaks, or setting aside a few minutes each day for mindfulness meditation can all contribute to self-care without requiring significant time commitments. By reframing self-care as a necessary investment in overall well-being, individuals can prioritize it and allocate time accordingly.

Guilt and Self-Worth

Another barrier to self-care is the feeling of guilt or the belief that one does not deserve to prioritize their own needs. Many individuals, especially caregivers or those in helping professions, may feel guilty for taking time for themselves when there are others depending on them.

To address this, individuals need to recognize that self-care is not selfish but rather a fundamental aspect of maintaining mental wellness. By prioritizing self-care, individuals become better equipped to care for others and perform their responsibilities effectively. It is important to challenge negative self-talk and cultivate self-compassion. Self-care should be seen as an act of self-love and self-preservation, rather than an indulgence.

Lack of Knowledge or Resources

A lack of knowledge or resources can also present barriers to self-care. Some individuals may not have access to information about different self-care practices or may not be aware of the resources available to support their well-being.

To overcome this barrier, it is important to educate oneself about the various self-care strategies and identify resources that are accessible. This can involve reading books, attending workshops, or seeking guidance from mental health professionals. Online platforms and mobile applications can also provide valuable guidance and support for self-care practices. By becoming informed about the options available, individuals can make informed choices and find strategies that work best for their specific needs and circumstances.

Cultural and Societal Factors

Cultural and societal factors can also pose challenges to self-care. Traditional cultural norms or societal expectations may prioritize the needs of others over one's own well-being. This can create a barrier for individuals who feel obligated to fulfill these expectations at the expense of their own self-care.

To address this, it is essential to challenge societal norms and cultivate a culture of self-care within communities and organizations. By promoting open conversations about the importance of self-care and the benefits it brings, individuals can support and encourage each other to prioritize their well-being. Additionally, cultural practices that promote self-care can be integrated and adapted to align with individual preferences and values.

Lack of Motivation or Willpower

Finally, a lack of motivation or willpower can be a significant barrier to implementing self-care practices. It can be challenging to make consistent and sustained efforts towards self-care, especially when faced with competing demands and responsibilities.

To overcome this barrier, individuals can start by setting realistic and achievable goals for self-care. Breaking down larger goals into smaller, manageable steps can make them more attainable. Seeking support from friends, family, or support groups can also provide motivation and accountability in maintaining self-care practices. It is important to remember that self-care is a journey, and setbacks or lapses should be seen as opportunities for growth and learning, rather than as failures.

In conclusion, while self-care is crucial for mental well-being, there are challenges and barriers that individuals may encounter. These barriers include time constraints, guilt and self-worth issues, lack of knowledge or resources, cultural and societal factors, and lack of motivation or willpower. By understanding and addressing these challenges, individuals can develop strategies to overcome them and make self-care a regular part of their lives. It is important to remember that self-care is a personal and individualized process, and finding what works best for oneself is key to achieving optimal mental wellness.

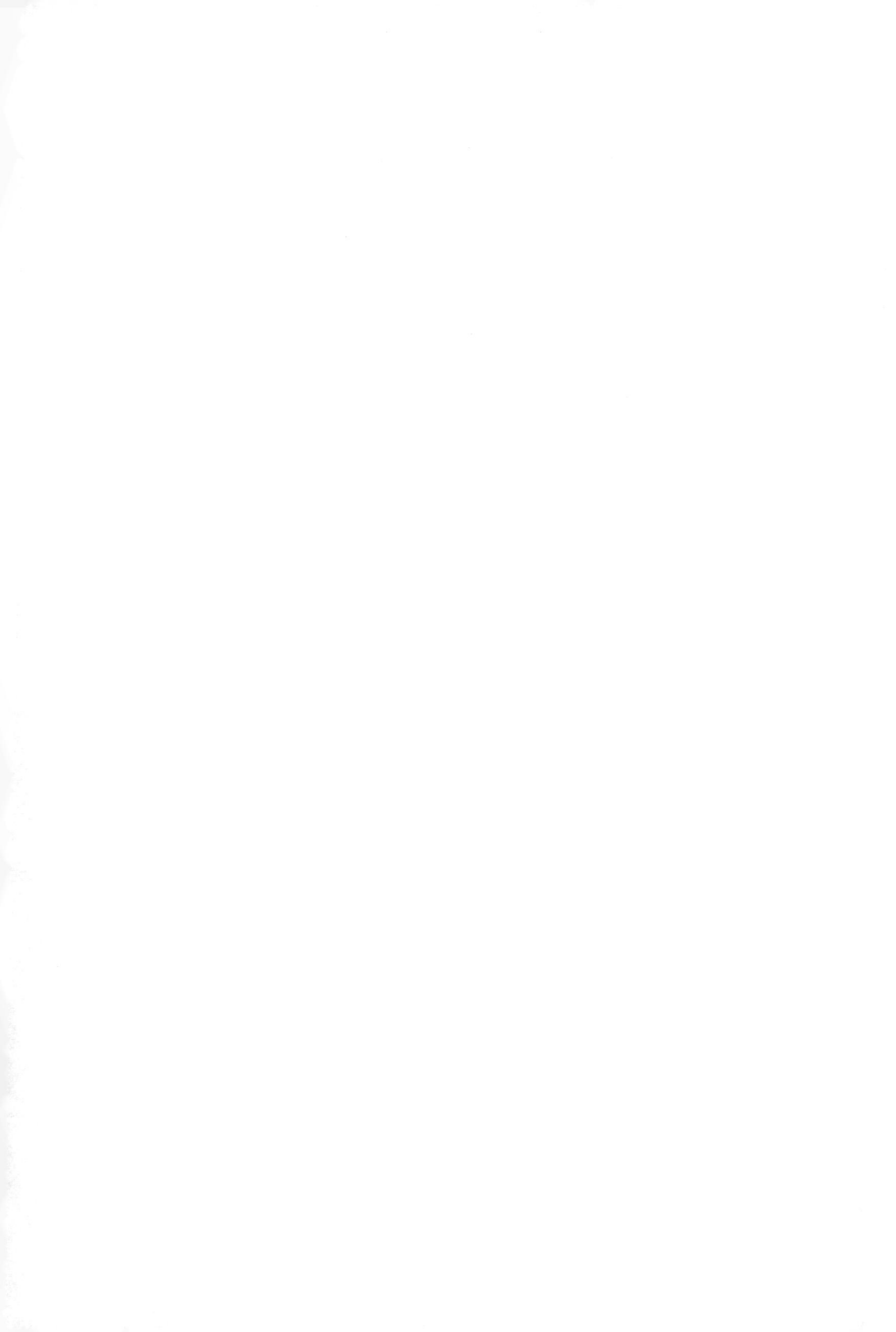

Cutting-Edge Research in Mental Health and Wellbeing

Advancements in Neuroscience and Mental Health

Introduction to Neuroscience and Its Role in Understanding Mental Health

Neuroscience, the study of the nervous system, has significantly contributed to our understanding of mental health and has revolutionized the field of psychiatry. By exploring the intricate workings of the brain and its connection to mental processes, researchers have uncovered valuable insights into the causes and mechanisms of various mental health disorders, leading to more effective treatments and interventions.

The Nervous System: The Foundation of Neuroscience

The nervous system is a complex network of cells, tissues, and organs that coordinate and regulate the body's functions and respond to internal and external stimuli. It is divided into two main components: the central nervous system (CNS) and the peripheral nervous system (PNS).

The CNS consists of the brain and spinal cord, while the PNS encompasses all the nerves that extend beyond the CNS, transmitting signals to and from the brain. The PNS can be further divided into the somatic nervous system, responsible for voluntary movements, and the autonomic nervous system, governing involuntary functions such as heartbeat and digestion.

Neurons: The Building Blocks of the Nervous System

At the core of the nervous system are specialized cells called neurons. Neurons are responsible for transmitting electrical and chemical signals throughout the body. They consist of three main parts: the cell body, dendrites, and an axon.

The cell body contains the nucleus and other essential cellular components. Dendrites are short, branched extensions that receive signals from other neurons and transmit them towards the cell body. The axon is a long, slender fiber that carries signals away from the cell body and transmits them to other neurons or target cells.

Neurotransmitters: Chemical Messengers of the Nervous System

Neurons communicate with each other through chemical signals called neurotransmitters. These molecules are released from the axon terminals of one neuron and bind to receptors on the dendrites or cell bodies of neighboring neurons, allowing for the transmission of signals across synapses.

Several neurotransmitters have been identified, each playing a unique role in regulating different aspects of behavior, cognition, and emotion. For example, serotonin is involved in mood regulation, dopamine is associated with reward and pleasure, and gamma-aminobutyric acid (GABA) inhibits the activity of neurons, promoting relaxation.

Brain Anatomy and Mental Health

The brain, the central organ of the nervous system, plays a crucial role in mental health. It consists of various structures, each responsible for specific functions. Understanding how these structures interact and contribute to mental processes is essential for comprehending mental health disorders.

The cerebral cortex, the outer layer of the brain, is responsible for higher-order functions such as cognition, perception, and decision-making. It is divided into lobes, each with its distinct functions. For example, the frontal lobe is involved in executive functions, the parietal lobe in sensory processing, the temporal lobe in auditory perception, and the occipital lobe in visual processing.

Other crucial structures include the limbic system, involved in emotions and memory, and the basal ganglia, responsible for motor control. The hypothalamus regulates bodily functions and hormone production, and the amygdala plays a vital role in processing emotions.

The Role of Neuroscience in Understanding Mental Health

Neuroscience has shed light on the neural underpinnings of mental health by investigating how abnormalities in brain structure and function contribute to the development and manifestation of mental health disorders. By studying the brain through various techniques such as neuroimaging and electrophysiology, researchers have made significant discoveries, shaping our understanding of these disorders.

For instance, studies have revealed differences in brain activation patterns between individuals with depression and those without, providing insight into the neural mechanisms underlying depressive symptoms. Additionally, research has shown that abnormalities in brain regions involved in fear processing contribute to the development of anxiety disorders.

Neuroscience has also elucidated the impact of genetics and environmental factors on mental health. Advances in molecular biology and genetics have allowed researchers to identify specific genes associated with certain mental health disorders. Furthermore, studies have shown that environmental factors, such as early-life experiences and trauma, can alter gene expression and increase the risk of developing mental health conditions.

Implications for Mental Health Treatment

The knowledge gained from neuroscience research has had a profound impact on the development of treatments for mental health disorders. By targeting the underlying neural mechanisms involved, therapies can be designed to address specific deficits or imbalances.

The use of psychopharmacological interventions, such as antidepressants or antipsychotics, aims to restore neurotransmitter balance and alleviate symptoms. Neurofeedback, a technique that allows individuals to self-regulate their brain activity, has shown promising results in conditions such as attention deficit hyperactivity disorder (ADHD) and post-traumatic stress disorder (PTSD).

Additionally, neuromodulation techniques, such as transcranial magnetic stimulation (TMS) and deep brain stimulation (DBS), involve applying electromagnetic or electrical stimulation to specific brain regions to modulate neural activity and alleviate symptoms.

Challenges and Future Directions

While neuroscience has made significant strides in understanding mental health, several challenges persist. The complexity of the brain and the intricate interactions between various neural circuits make it challenging to fully comprehend the underlying mechanisms of mental health disorders.

Furthermore, ethical considerations, such as ensuring the privacy and autonomy of individuals participating in research studies, are of utmost importance in neuroscience research. Striking a balance between advancing knowledge and safeguarding human rights and dignity is a continuous endeavor.

Looking ahead, emerging techniques, such as optogenetics, which involves using light to control neural activity, and advances in artificial intelligence, hold great promise for further unraveling the mysteries of the brain and advancing our understanding of mental health.

Summary

Neuroscience serves as a cornerstone in our understanding of mental health. By delving into the intricate workings of the nervous system and exploring the brain's inner workings, researchers have made groundbreaking progress in unraveling the causes and mechanisms underlying mental health disorders. This knowledge has paved the way for more effective and personalized treatments, improving the lives of individuals living with mental health conditions. As neuroscience continues to advance, it holds the potential to shape the future of mental health and well-being, offering hope for better outcomes and greater understanding.

Neuroimaging Techniques in Mental Health Research

Neuroimaging techniques have revolutionized the field of mental health research by providing detailed insights into the structure, function, and connectivity of the brain. These techniques help us understand the underlying neural mechanisms involved in various mental health disorders and provide valuable information for diagnostic purposes, treatment planning, and monitoring therapeutic interventions. In this section, we will explore the different neuroimaging techniques used in mental health research and their applications.

Structural Imaging

Structural imaging techniques allow us to visualize the anatomy of the brain, providing information about its size, shape, and structural abnormalities. Magnetic Resonance Imaging (MRI) is the most commonly used structural imaging technique in mental health research. MRI uses a strong magnetic field and radio waves to produce high-resolution images of the brain. It can help identify structural abnormalities such as tumors, lesions, or changes in brain volume associated with mental health disorders.

For example, researchers have used MRI to study the hippocampus, a brain region involved in memory and emotion regulation, in individuals with post-traumatic stress disorder (PTSD). They have found that the volume of the hippocampus is often reduced in individuals with PTSD, suggesting a link between trauma exposure, stress, and structural changes in the brain.

Functional Imaging

Functional imaging techniques allow us to observe brain activity in real-time. These techniques provide valuable insights into the underlying neural processes associated with various mental health disorders. Positron Emission Tomography (PET) and functional Magnetic Resonance Imaging (fMRI) are commonly used functional imaging techniques in mental health research.

PET imaging involves injecting a radioactive substance into the bloodstream, which is then absorbed by the brain. By measuring the emitted radiation, PET can identify areas of increased or decreased brain activity, highlighting areas of abnormal function. PET has been used to study conditions such as schizophrenia, depression, and addiction, revealing alterations in brain function that correlate with these disorders.

On the other hand, fMRI measures changes in blood flow in the brain, which is an indirect marker of neural activity. By detecting these changes, fMRI can identify brain regions that are activated or deactivated during specific tasks or resting states. This technique has been instrumental in understanding the functional connectivity within neural networks and identifying aberrant connectivity patterns in mental health disorders. For instance, fMRI studies have shown altered functional connectivity in individuals with autism spectrum disorder (ASD), providing insights into the social and cognitive deficits associated with the condition.

Diffusion Imaging

Diffusion imaging techniques, such as Diffusion Tensor Imaging (DTI), enable us to study the white matter tracts in the brain. White matter consists of bundles of nerve fibers that facilitate communication between different brain regions. DTI measures the movement of water molecules along these fibers and provides information about the structural integrity and organization of white matter tracts.

DTI has been used to investigate conditions such as traumatic brain injury, multiple sclerosis, and schizophrenia, revealing disruptions in white matter connectivity. For example, in individuals with schizophrenia, DTI studies have shown reduced integrity of white matter tracts connecting frontal and temporal brain regions, which may underlie cognitive and perceptual abnormalities associated with the disorder.

Limitations and Future Directions

While neuroimaging techniques have greatly advanced our understanding of mental health disorders, there are some limitations to consider. The cost and availability of advanced imaging equipment can be a barrier for many researchers and clinicians. Additionally, the interpretation of neuroimaging findings requires expertise in image analysis and a nuanced understanding of the limitations of these techniques.

Looking ahead, there are exciting possibilities for the integration of neuroimaging with other technologies such as virtual reality and machine learning. Virtual reality can provide immersive environments for studying psychiatric symptoms, while machine learning algorithms can help analyze large datasets and identify biomarkers for mental health disorders.

In conclusion, neuroimaging techniques have transformed the field of mental health research by allowing us to investigate the structure, function, and connectivity of the brain. Structural imaging, functional imaging, and diffusion imaging provide valuable insights into the underlying neural mechanisms of mental health disorders. However, challenges remain in terms of accessibility and interpretation of neuroimaging findings. With continued advancements and interdisciplinary collaborations, neuroimaging holds great promise in shaping the future of mental health research and personalized treatment approaches.

Emerging Findings and Implications for Treatment

In recent years, there have been significant advancements in the field of mental health research, leading to emerging findings that have the potential to transform the way we approach treatment. These findings offer new insights into the underlying mechanisms of mental health disorders and provide innovative strategies for intervention and support. In this section, we will explore some of these emerging findings and their implications for treatment.

Understanding the Complexity of Mental Health Disorders

One of the key emerging findings in mental health research is the recognition of the complexity of mental health disorders. Traditionally, mental health disorders have been categorized based on specific symptoms or diagnostic criteria. However, research has shown that mental health disorders are heterogeneous in nature, with significant variation in symptom presentation, underlying neural mechanisms, and treatment response.

Emerging findings highlight the importance of adopting a personalized approach to treatment, taking into account individual differences in symptomatology, genetics, environmental factors, and treatment preferences. By recognizing the complexity of mental health disorders, healthcare professionals can tailor interventions to meet the unique needs of each individual, leading to more effective and targeted treatment outcomes.

Advancements in Neuroimaging Techniques

Neuroimaging techniques, such as functional magnetic resonance imaging (fMRI) and positron emission tomography (PET), have revolutionized our understanding of the brain and its role in mental health disorders. These techniques allow researchers to visualize and study the structure, function, and connectivity of the brain in unprecedented detail.

Emerging findings from neuroimaging research have provided valuable insights into the neurobiological basis of mental health disorders, identifying specific brain regions and neural networks that are implicated in various psychiatric conditions. For example, studies have shown that individuals with depression exhibit decreased activity in the prefrontal cortex, a region involved in emotional regulation and cognitive control.

These findings have significant implications for treatment. By targeting specific brain regions and neural circuits implicated in mental health disorders, interventions can be designed to modulate neural activity and restore normal functioning. Techniques such as transcranial magnetic stimulation (TMS) and deep brain stimulation (DBS) have emerged as potential treatment options that directly target brain regions associated with psychiatric symptoms.

Exploring the Gut-Brain Axis

Another emerging area of research with profound implications for mental health treatment is the study of the gut-brain axis. The gut and the brain are connected through a bidirectional communication system, with the microbiota in the gut influencing brain function and vice versa.

Research has shown that imbalances in gut microbiota, collectively known as dysbiosis, are associated with various mental health disorders, including depression, anxiety, and autism spectrum disorders. These findings point to the potential of interventions targeting the gut microbiota as a novel treatment approach.

Probiotics, prebiotics, and dietary interventions aimed at modulating the gut microbiota have shown promise in reducing symptoms of mental health disorders. For example, certain strains of probiotics have been found to alleviate symptoms of depression and anxiety by producing neurotransmitters and anti-inflammatory compounds.

However, it is important to note that the gut-brain axis is still a relatively new area of research, and further studies are needed to better understand the complex interactions between the gut microbiota and mental health. Nonetheless, these emerging findings open up new possibilities for the development of innovative and personalized treatment approaches.

Considering the Role of Social Determinants

Emerging research emphasizes the significant impact of social determinants on mental health outcomes. Social determinants refer to the economic, social, and environmental factors that shape an individual's health and wellbeing. Factors such as poverty, discrimination, social support, and access to healthcare can profoundly influence mental health.

Studies have shown that individuals from disadvantaged backgrounds are more likely to experience mental health disorders due to increased exposure to chronic stressors and limited access to resources. Additionally, social support has been identified as a protective factor against mental health disorders, highlighting the importance of strong social connections in promoting wellbeing.

The recognition of the role of social determinants in mental health has led to a shift towards a more holistic and comprehensive approach to treatment. It becomes crucial to consider not only the individual's symptoms but also the broader social and environmental context in which they exist. This perspective allows for the development of interventions that address the root causes of mental health disorders and promote resilience and wellbeing.

Integrating Technology into Treatment

Advancements in technology have also made a significant impact on mental health treatment. Mobile applications, wearable devices, and online platforms have transformed the way individuals access information, support, and intervention for mental health disorders.

Emerging findings suggest that technology-driven interventions have the potential to improve access to mental health care, enhance treatment effectiveness, and reduce barriers to care. For example, smartphone apps that provide cognitive-behavioral therapy (CBT) exercises or mindfulness-based interventions can empower individuals to actively engage in self-management and monitor their progress.

Virtual reality (VR) and augmented reality (AR) technologies have also shown promise in the treatment of various mental health disorders. VR-based exposure therapy has been used successfully in the treatment of phobias and post-traumatic stress disorder (PTSD), allowing individuals to confront their fears in a controlled and safe environment.

However, it is essential to consider the limitations and potential risks associated with the use of technology in mental health treatment. Privacy concerns, the digital divide, and the need for human connection and therapeutic rapport must be carefully addressed to ensure the ethical and effective integration of technology into mental health care.

Conclusion

The emerging findings in mental health research provide exciting opportunities for the transformation of mental health treatment. By embracing the complexity of mental health disorders, leveraging advancements in neuroimaging, exploring the gut-brain axis, considering social determinants, and integrating technology into treatment, we can develop innovative, personalized, and effective interventions that improve the lives of individuals with mental health disorders.

As the field continues to evolve, it is essential to encourage continued research, collaboration, and innovation. By prioritizing research that embraces the principles of diversity, equity, and inclusion, we can work towards a future where mental health care is accessible, effective, and truly transformative.

Innovative Technologies in Mental Health Care

Telehealth and Telemedicine in Mental Health

Telehealth and telemedicine have emerged as innovative and transformative approaches in the field of mental health. With advancements in technology and the increasing demand for accessible and convenient healthcare services, telehealth has gained significant attention as a viable solution for improving mental health outcomes. In this section, we will explore the various aspects of telehealth and telemedicine in the context of mental health, including its definition, applications, benefits, challenges, and future directions.

Definition of Telehealth and Telemedicine

Telehealth refers to the delivery of healthcare services, including mental health services, using telecommunication technologies. It involves the remote diagnosis, treatment, monitoring, and general support for patients who are located in different geographical locations from their healthcare providers. Telemedicine, on the other hand, specifically focuses on the delivery of medical services through telecommunication technologies. While the scope of telehealth is broader, telemedicine is a subset of telehealth that centers on clinical care.

In the context of mental health, telehealth and telemedicine enable mental health professionals to provide counseling, therapy, assessment, and other mental health support remotely. These services are delivered through various means, such as video conferences, phone calls, text-based messaging, and mobile applications. Telehealth and telemedicine platforms may also incorporate other functionalities, such as secure messaging, electronic health record management, and remote monitoring of vital signs and symptoms.

Applications of Telehealth and Telemedicine in Mental Health

Telehealth and telemedicine have been widely applied in various areas of mental health care. They have proven to be effective and efficient in delivering mental health services, especially in situations where face-to-face interactions are challenging or not readily available. Some key applications include:

1. **Remote Counseling and Therapy:** Telehealth enables mental health professionals to provide counseling and therapy sessions remotely. This is particularly beneficial for individuals who have limited physical mobility, live in rural or remote areas, or prefer the convenience and privacy of online sessions. It also allows for immediate access to mental health support during times of crisis or emergencies.

2. **Psychiatric Consultations:** Telemedicine facilitates remote psychiatric consultations, where individuals can connect with psychiatrists or other mental health specialists through video conferencing. This is particularly useful in areas with a shortage of mental health professionals or when immediate consultations are needed for complex cases.

3. **Screening and Assessment:** Telehealth platforms can be used for remote screening and assessment of mental health conditions. Through secure online questionnaires and assessments, individuals can provide relevant information to mental health professionals, who can then make informed diagnoses and treatment recommendations.

4. **Support Groups and Peer Counseling:** Telehealth provides opportunities for virtual support groups and peer counseling sessions. Individuals facing similar mental health challenges can connect and interact in online communities, offering support, empathy, and shared experiences.

5. **Education and Training:** Telehealth platforms enable mental health professionals to provide education and training sessions remotely. This benefits both professionals seeking continuing education and training and individuals interested in learning more about mental health and self-care techniques.

Benefits of Telehealth and Telemedicine

The implementation of telehealth and telemedicine in mental health care offers a wide range of benefits, both for patients and mental health professionals.

Improved Access to Care: One of the primary advantages of telehealth is the increased accessibility to mental health services, particularly for underserved populations. It eliminates geographical barriers, making mental health care available to individuals residing in remote or rural areas where mental health services may be limited or unavailable. It also reduces the burden of traveling long distances, especially for those with limited mobility or transportation options.

Convenience and Flexibility: Telehealth provides convenience and flexibility in accessing mental health care. Patients can schedule appointments at their preferred time and receive services from the comfort of their own homes. This is particularly beneficial for individuals with busy schedules, caregivers, or those who may experience anxiety or discomfort in traditional clinical settings.

Privacy and Confidentiality: Telehealth offers increased privacy and confidentiality compared to in-person visits. Individuals can have therapy sessions or consultations in a secure and familiar environment, minimizing the risk of being seen or recognized by others in a waiting room. Additionally, telehealth platforms ensure secure data transmission and storage, maintaining the confidentiality of sensitive patient information.

Cost-Effectiveness: Telehealth and telemedicine have the potential to reduce healthcare costs for both patients and healthcare systems. It eliminates the need for transportation expenses, reduces missed workdays, and minimizes other costs associated with in-person visits. For healthcare systems, telehealth can help optimize resource allocation and reduce the strain on physical infrastructure.

Continuity of Care: Telehealth enables seamless and continuous care, particularly in situations where face-to-face visits are not feasible. It allows for regular check-ins, follow-ups, and ongoing support, ensuring that individuals receive consistent care throughout their mental health journey. This continuity contributes to better treatment outcomes and reduces the risk of relapse.

Challenges and Considerations

While telehealth and telemedicine hold great promise for mental health care, several challenges and considerations need to be addressed for their successful implementation.

Technological Barriers: Adequate access to technology and reliable internet connection are essential for telehealth services. However, some individuals may lack access to the necessary devices or have limited internet connectivity, particularly in marginalized or low-income communities. Efforts must be made to bridge the digital divide and ensure equitable access to telehealth services.

Security and Privacy Concerns: Maintaining the security and privacy of patient data is critical in telehealth. Health systems and mental health professionals must adopt robust data protection measures to safeguard patient information from unauthorized access or breaches. Compliance with relevant privacy regulations and standards is essential for ensuring trust and confidence in telehealth services.

Reliance on Technology: The reliance on technology for telehealth services introduces the risk of technical failures or disruptions. Power outages, internet outages, or technical glitches can interrupt sessions and impact the quality of care. Backup plans and contingency measures should be in place to address such situations and minimize their impact on patient care.

Loss of Nonverbal Cues: Telehealth platforms may not capture all nonverbal cues, which can be essential in mental health assessments and interventions. Mental health professionals must be trained to adapt their approaches in a telehealth setting and make the most of the available cues and information. Additionally, technology advancements should aim to enhance the transmission of nonverbal cues for more accurate assessment and treatment.

Ethical and Legal Considerations: Telehealth raises ethical and legal considerations that must be carefully addressed. These include obtaining informed consent, ensuring appropriate boundaries, maintaining confidentiality, and handling emergency situations or crisis interventions remotely. Mental health professionals must adhere to relevant ethical guidelines and legal frameworks specific to telehealth practice.

Future Directions

The future of telehealth and telemedicine in mental health holds great potential for further advancements and integration into standard care practices. Some areas of future development include:

Technological Innovations: Continued advancements in technology will shape the telehealth landscape. This includes the development of more user-friendly platforms, enhanced video and audio quality, improved data security measures, and increased interoperability with electronic health records and other healthcare systems.

Artificial Intelligence (AI) and Machine Learning: AI and machine learning algorithms can be integrated into telehealth platforms to enhance screening, assessments, and treatment planning. These technologies can help automate certain processes, identify patterns, and provide personalized recommendations to mental health professionals and individuals seeking care.

Virtual Reality (VR) and Augmented Reality (AR): VR and AR technologies have the potential to revolutionize mental health care by enabling immersive and interactive interventions. Virtual environments can be created for exposure therapy, relaxation techniques, and even social skills training. These technologies may provide a more engaging and effective means of delivering therapy remotely.

Integration with Wearable Devices: Telehealth can be integrated with wearable devices to monitor individuals' mental health in real-time. Wearable devices, such as smartwatches or biosensors, can collect data on physiological indicators (e.g., heart rate, sleep patterns) and provide valuable insights to mental health professionals for assessments and treatment planning.

Telehealth in Crisis Intervention: Telehealth can play a crucial role in crisis intervention and suicide prevention. Crisis helplines and suicide prevention hotlines can utilize telehealth platforms to provide immediate support and interventions. Integration with emergency services and resources can ensure timely access to critical care.

Overall, telehealth and telemedicine have the potential to transform mental health care delivery by increasing accessibility, improving convenience, and enhancing continuity of care. However, careful attention must be given to addressing technological, ethical, and legal considerations to ensure the responsible and effective implementation of these approaches. Continued research, innovation, and collaboration will shape the future of telehealth in mental health, ultimately leading to better mental health outcomes for individuals worldwide.

Exercises

1. Research and explain the legal and regulatory considerations for practicing telehealth and telemedicine in your country or region. What licenses or certifications are required for mental health professionals to provide services through telehealth?

2. In rural or remote areas where internet connectivity may be limited, what alternative telehealth strategies can be implemented to ensure accessibility to mental health care?

3. Discuss the potential benefits and challenges of using virtual reality-based therapy for individuals with phobias or anxiety disorders. How can telehealth platforms integrate virtual reality technologies to deliver these interventions?

4. Explore the ethical implications of providing therapy or counseling services remotely through telehealth platforms. What are the potential ethical dilemmas that mental health professionals may face, and how can they be addressed?

Resources

- American Telemedicine Association: https://www.americantelemed.org/
- Telehealth Resource Centers: https://www.telehealthresourcecenter.org/
- National Consortium of Telehealth Resource Centers: https://www.telehealthresourcecenter.org/learn/telehealthbasics/

Further Reading

- Bashshur, R. L., Shannon, G. W., Bashshur, N., Yellowlees, P. M., & Ranganathan, C. (2015). The empirical evidence for telemedicine interventions in mental disorders. Telemedicine Journal and e-Health, 21(12), 987-992.
- Shore, J. H., Yellowlees, P., & Caudill, R. (2018). Telepsychiatry and Health Technologies: A Guide for Mental Health Professionals. American Psychiatric Association Publishing.

- Hilty, D. M., Chan, S., Torous, J., Mahabalagiri, V., & Das, S. (2020). Roles of psychiatrists and other mental health professionals in team-based treatment using telepsychiatry and digital technologies. The Journal of Clinical Psychiatry, 81(2), 19com13312.

This concludes our exploration of telehealth and telemedicine in mental health. In the next section, we will delve into the realm of virtual reality and augmented reality as transformative tools in mental health therapy.

Virtual Reality and Augmented Reality in Therapy

Virtual Reality (VR) and Augmented Reality (AR) are innovative technologies that have gained significant attention in various fields, including mental health care. They offer unique opportunities to create immersive and interactive experiences that can be tailored to meet the specific needs of individuals seeking therapy. In this section, we will explore the applications of VR and AR in therapy, their benefits and challenges, and their potential to revolutionize mental health treatment.

Introduction to Virtual Reality and Augmented Reality

Virtual Reality is a technology that uses computer-generated simulations to create a three-dimensional environment that feels realistic and immersive. It usually involves wearing a head-mounted display (HMD) that tracks the user's head movements, allowing them to explore and interact with the virtual environment. Augmented Reality, on the other hand, overlays virtual elements onto the real world, enhancing it with digital content that can be viewed through a device such as a smartphone or smart glasses.

Both VR and AR have the potential to transform therapy by providing a safe and controlled environment for individuals to practice skills, confront fears, and process traumatic experiences. By creating simulations that replicate real-world scenarios or trigger specific emotions, therapists can guide clients through therapeutic interventions in a more engaging and effective way.

Applications of VR and AR in Therapy

1. Exposure Therapy: One of the most prominent applications of VR in therapy is exposure therapy, which involves exposing individuals to anxiety-provoking stimuli in a controlled environment. VR can simulate these stimuli, such as heights, public speaking, or flying, allowing individuals to gradually and safely confront their fears.

By providing a sense of presence and immersion, VR enables therapists to create realistic and personalized exposure scenarios, enhancing the effectiveness of the treatment.

2. Post-Traumatic Stress Disorder (PTSD) Treatment: VR has shown promising results in the treatment of PTSD. It can recreate traumatic events or environments, allowing individuals to process and desensitize traumatic memories in a safe space. Therapists can use VR to guide clients through virtual scenarios, helping them confront and gradually reduce their distressing symptoms.

3. Social Skills Training: VR and AR can be valuable tools for individuals with social anxiety or autism spectrum disorders. These technologies can simulate social interactions and provide individuals with opportunities to practice social skills in a controlled and supportive environment. By experimenting with different scenarios and receiving feedback, individuals can improve their social competence and reduce anxiety in real-world social situations.

4. Pain Management: VR has shown promise in alleviating pain and discomfort by creating immersive and engaging experiences. By distracting individuals from their physical sensations, VR can reduce pain perception and improve overall well-being. Additionally, AR can be used as a complementary tool in pain management, providing real-time information and visualizations to help individuals understand and manage their pain.

Benefits and Challenges of VR and AR in Therapy

The use of VR and AR in therapy offers several advantages:

1. Enhanced Immersion: VR and AR technologies provide a high level of immersion, allowing individuals to feel present in the virtual environment or augmented reality experience. This sense of presence can enhance engagement and the effectiveness of therapeutic interventions.

2. Safety and Control: Virtual simulations provide a safe and controlled environment for individuals to practice skills or confront fears. Therapists can customize the virtual scenarios to the individual's needs, gradually increasing the level of difficulty or exposure, ensuring a comfortable and controlled experience.

3. Ecological Validity: VR and AR can offer more ecological validity compared to traditional therapy settings. The ability to recreate real-world situations and experiences makes therapy more relevant and applicable to everyday life.

Despite these benefits, there are also challenges associated with the use of VR and AR in therapy:

1. Cost and Accessibility: VR and AR technology can be costly, especially for high-quality systems. Additionally, not everyone may have access to the necessary

equipment or expertise to use these technologies effectively.

2. Technical Limitations: VR and AR technologies are still evolving, and there may be limitations in terms of graphics quality, motion sickness, or device compatibility. Overcoming these technical challenges is crucial to ensure a smooth and comfortable user experience.

3. Ethical Considerations: The use of VR and AR in therapy raises ethical concerns, such as ensuring informed consent, protecting privacy, and avoiding potential harm. Therapists must be mindful of these ethical considerations and follow ethical guidelines when using these technologies in practice.

Future Directions and Conclusion

The future of VR and AR in therapy looks promising, with ongoing research and development aiming to address the current challenges and expand the applications of these technologies. Advancements in technology, such as improved graphics quality and more affordable devices, will increase accessibility and usability.

Furthermore, the combination of VR and AR with other emerging technologies, such as artificial intelligence and biofeedback systems, holds great potential for personalized and interactive therapy approaches. These technologies can provide real-time feedback, adaptive interventions, and data-driven insights, enhancing the effectiveness and efficiency of therapy.

In conclusion, VR and AR have the potential to revolutionize mental health treatment by providing immersive and interactive experiences that can be customized to individual needs. While there are challenges to overcome, the benefits of these technologies in exposure therapy, PTSD treatment, social skills training, and pain management are promising. As research and development in this field continue to progress, the integration of VR and AR into mainstream mental health care practices may become more widespread, offering new possibilities for therapy and improving the lives of individuals experiencing mental health challenges.

Wearable Devices and Apps for Mental Health Monitoring and Support

Advancements in technology have revolutionized various aspects of healthcare, including mental health. Wearable devices and smartphone apps have emerged as powerful tools for monitoring and supporting mental health. These innovative technologies provide individuals with the ability to track their mental well-being and access support in real-time, promoting self-awareness and proactive management of mental health conditions. In this section, we will explore the role of wearable devices and apps in mental health monitoring and support, their benefits, challenges, and future prospects.

The Role of Wearable Devices in Mental Health

Wearable devices, such as smartwatches and fitness trackers, have gained popularity in recent years for their ability to monitor various aspects of physical health. However, these devices also have significant potential for monitoring mental health. By utilizing sensors and advanced algorithms, wearable devices can collect data on physiological and behavioral patterns that are indicative of mental well-being.

One key application of wearable devices in mental health is the monitoring of stress levels. These devices can measure physiological indicators, such as heart rate variability and skin conductance, which provide insights into the body's response to stress. By continuously tracking stress levels throughout the day, individuals can identify triggers and make necessary lifestyle adjustments to manage stress effectively.

Wearable devices can also monitor sleep patterns, which have a profound impact on mental health. Sleep disturbances are common in various mental health disorders, and tracking sleep quality can provide valuable information for both individuals and healthcare professionals. By analyzing sleep duration, efficiency, and stages, wearable devices can help identify sleep problems and guide interventions for improved sleep hygiene.

The Role of Apps in Mental Health Support

In addition to wearable devices, smartphone apps play a vital role in mental health support. These apps offer a range of functionalities, from providing psychoeducation and coping strategies to connecting individuals with mental health professionals and support communities. The convenience and accessibility of smartphone apps make them highly suitable for delivering mental health interventions.

Many apps leverage evidence-based therapeutic approaches to address specific mental health challenges. For instance, cognitive-behavioral therapy (CBT) apps provide users with tools and techniques to identify and modify negative thought patterns. These apps often include interactive exercises, mood tracking features, and journaling capabilities to assist individuals in managing their mental health on a day-to-day basis.

Apps also enable remote monitoring and support from mental health professionals. Through secure messaging platforms and virtual therapy sessions, individuals can receive real-time guidance and feedback, particularly beneficial for those who face barriers to in-person care, such as geographical or financial limitations. Additionally, apps that connect users to peer support networks foster a sense of community and reduce feelings of isolation.

Benefits and Challenges of Wearable Devices and Apps

The integration of wearable devices and apps in mental health monitoring and support offers several benefits. Firstly, these technologies empower individuals to actively participate in their mental health management. By providing real-time data and personalized feedback, individuals gain a better understanding of their mental well-being and can make more informed decisions regarding their lifestyle choices and treatment plans.

Wearable devices and apps also have the potential to enhance communication and collaboration between individuals and healthcare professionals. The data collected by these technologies can facilitate more accurate assessments, as healthcare providers have access to a comprehensive overview of an individual's mental health status. This can lead to more personalized treatment recommendations and improved outcomes.

However, several challenges need to be addressed to maximize the effectiveness of wearable devices and apps in mental health. Firstly, privacy and data security concerns must be adequately addressed to ensure that individuals' sensitive information remains protected. Clear guidelines and regulations regarding data collection, storage, and sharing need to be in place to build trust and safeguard confidentiality.

Moreover, the accuracy and reliability of wearable devices and apps should be carefully evaluated. Calibration and validation studies are necessary to ensure that these technologies provide accurate measurements and produce reliable data. Additionally, addressing issues of user engagement and adherence is crucial to ensure long-term usage and sustained benefits.

Future Prospects

The future of wearable devices and apps in mental health looks promising, with several exciting developments on the horizon. As technology continues to evolve, wearable devices are becoming more sophisticated, offering additional features such as electroencephalography (EEG) for monitoring brain activity and detecting mental states. These advancements can provide deeper insights into mental health and aid in the development of targeted interventions.

Furthermore, the integration of artificial intelligence (AI) holds tremendous potential for enhancing the capabilities of wearable devices and apps. AI algorithms can analyze vast amounts of data, identify patterns, and make personalized predictions, thereby enabling more precise and tailored interventions. For example, AI-based chatbots can offer immediate support and guidance to individuals in distress, complementing traditional therapy.

To fully realize the potential of wearable devices and apps, interdisciplinary collaborations and partnerships between technology developers, mental health professionals, and researchers are essential. The involvement of diverse stakeholders can ensure that these technologies are evidence-based, user-friendly, and culturally sensitive. Additionally, increased investment in research and development can drive innovation in this field and lead to novel solutions for mental health monitoring and support.

In conclusion, wearable devices and apps have become valuable tools for mental health monitoring and support. They empower individuals to take an active role in their mental well-being, provide access to evidence-based interventions, and foster collaborations between individuals and healthcare professionals. While challenges exist, the future holds exciting prospects for the further integration of these technologies, ultimately shaping a transformed landscape of mental health care.

Psychedelic-Assisted Therapy

History and Revival of Psychedelic-Assisted Therapy

Psychedelic-assisted therapy has a long and fascinating history, marked by periods of both popularity and controversy. In this section, we will explore the origins of psychedelic-assisted therapy, its decline, and its recent revival as a promising treatment approach for mental health disorders.

Origins of Psychedelic-Assisted Therapy

The use of psychedelics for therapeutic purposes can be traced back to indigenous cultures that have long incorporated these substances into their healing practices. For example, indigenous tribes in the Amazon rainforest have been using ayahuasca, a psychedelic brew, as a spiritual and medicinal tool for centuries. Similarly, Native American tribes have used peyote, a psychedelic cactus, in their religious ceremonies.

The modern era of psychedelic-assisted therapy began in the mid-20th century with the discovery of lysergic acid diethylamide (LSD) by Swiss chemist Albert Hofmann in 1943. Following its accidental ingestion, Hofmann experienced vivid hallucinations and altered perception, leading to further investigation of the substance's potential therapeutic effects.

Psychedelics gained significant attention in the 1950s and 1960s, with researchers exploring their potential applications in various fields, including psychiatry. Notable figures such as psychiatrists Humphry Osmond and Stanislav Grof conducted pioneering research on the therapeutic use of psychedelics, particularly LSD, in addressing mental health issues.

The Decline of Psychedelic-Assisted Therapy

Despite initial optimism, the widespread use of psychedelics in both therapeutic and non-therapeutic settings led to public concern and subsequent government crackdowns. In the mid-1960s, the counterculture movement and recreational use of psychedelics became associated with social unrest and public safety risks. This led to the criminalization of psychedelics and a halt in scientific research into their therapeutic potential.

As a result of these regulatory restrictions and societal backlash, psychedelic-assisted therapy was largely abandoned by the medical and psychiatric communities. The promising findings and potential benefits of early research were overshadowed by the negative portrayal of psychedelics in the media and political discourse.

Revival of Psychedelic-Assisted Therapy

In recent years, there has been a resurgence of interest in the therapeutic use of psychedelics. This revival can be attributed to several factors, including advancements in scientific research, shifts in societal attitudes, and the recognition of the limitations of traditional psychiatric treatments.

Scientific research has played a crucial role in rekindling interest in psychedelic-assisted therapy. Studies conducted in the late 20th century, such as those by psychiatrist Rick Doblin, demonstrated the potential benefits of psychedelics in treating conditions like post-traumatic stress disorder (PTSD) and anxiety. These findings, coupled with advancements in neuroscience and neuroimaging technologies, have provided a better understanding of the mechanisms of action underlying psychedelic therapy.

Another contributing factor to the revival of psychedelic-assisted therapy is a change in societal attitudes towards psychedelics. The decriminalization and legalization of psychedelic substances in certain jurisdictions have opened up avenues for further research and exploration. Additionally, public opinion has shifted, with growing recognition of the potential therapeutic benefits of psychedelics.

Furthermore, the limitations of traditional psychiatric treatments have led to an increased interest in alternative and complementary approaches. Traditional medications, such as antidepressants, often have limited effectiveness or significant side effects for some individuals. Psychedelic-assisted therapy offers a novel and potentially transformative treatment option that can complement existing therapeutic approaches.

Current Research and Future Directions

The recent resurgence in psychedelic-assisted therapy has sparked a wave of new research and clinical trials. Studies have explored the use of psychedelics, such as psilocybin (found in "magic mushrooms") and MDMA (also known as ecstasy), in treating a range of mental health conditions, including depression, PTSD, addiction, and end-of-life distress.

The results of several clinical trials have been promising, demonstrating significant improvements in symptoms and overall well-being. For example, studies using psilocybin-assisted therapy have shown remarkable efficacy in reducing depression and anxiety in individuals with treatment-resistant depression. Similarly, MDMA-assisted psychotherapy has shown promising results in alleviating PTSD symptoms.

However, it is important to note that psychedelic-assisted therapy is still in its early stages, and more research is needed to fully understand its potential benefits, risks, and long-term effects. Ethical considerations, safety protocols, and standardized treatment guidelines are crucial aspects that need to be addressed as this field continues to evolve.

In conclusion, the history of psychedelic-assisted therapy has witnessed both periods of promise and periods of controversy. The recent revival of interest in this therapeutic approach can be attributed to advancements in scientific research, changes in societal attitudes, and the limitations of traditional psychiatric treatments. As research in this field continues to expand, psychedelic-assisted therapy holds significant potential to transform the way we approach mental health treatment and improve the lives of individuals struggling with various mental health disorders.

Research on the Use of Psychedelics in Mental Health Treatment

The use of psychedelics in mental health treatment has gained significant attention in recent years. Researchers and clinicians have been exploring the potential therapeutic benefits of substances such as psilocybin (found in certain mushrooms), LSD, and MDMA (commonly known as ecstasy) in addressing various mental health conditions. This section will delve into the current state of research on the use of psychedelics in mental health treatment, including its history, efficacy, safety concerns, and future directions.

Historical Context

Psychedelic substances have a long-standing history of use in various cultures for spiritual, healing, and ceremonial purposes. However, their clinical use declined following their classification as Schedule I drugs in the 1970s, which restricted their research and clinical applications. In recent years, there has been a resurgence of interest, with researchers seeking to systematically explore their therapeutic potential.

Efficacy in Mental Health Treatment

The preliminary research on psychedelics suggests promising results in the treatment of certain mental health disorders. Studies have shown that psilocybin-assisted therapy can be effective in reducing symptoms of treatment-resistant depression, anxiety in patients with life-threatening illnesses, and tobacco, alcohol, and opioid addiction. Similarly, MDMA-assisted psychotherapy has shown promise in the treatment of post-traumatic stress disorder (PTSD) and is currently undergoing advanced trials for potential approval by regulatory bodies.

Mechanisms of Action

The mechanisms of action underlying the therapeutic effects of psychedelics are not fully understood. However, current research suggests that these substances modulate brain networks involved in mood regulation, emotional processing, and self-reflective awareness. Additionally, they may promote neuroplasticity and enhance the formation of new neural connections, which may contribute to long-term positive changes in mental health.

Safety Considerations

Safety is a critical aspect of any therapeutic intervention. While psychedelics have been shown to have a relatively low physiological toxicity profile, there are still considerations regarding their use. Psychedelic-assisted therapy should always be conducted in a controlled and supervised setting to ensure the physical and psychological well-being of participants. Additionally, appropriate screening processes, informed consent, and holistic integration support are essential components of ensuring patient safety.

Integration with Traditional Therapeutic Approaches

The use of psychedelics in mental health treatment is often integrated with traditional therapeutic approaches, such as psychotherapy. The psychedelic experience itself is seen as an adjunct to therapy, providing a catalyst for deep introspection, emotional release, and transformative insights. Following the psychedelic experience, therapists work with patients to integrate these insights into their daily lives, supporting sustained positive changes.

Challenges and Ethical Considerations

The use of psychedelics in therapy also presents several challenges and ethical considerations. These substances have the potential for misuse or recreational use, underscoring the need for careful regulation and professional supervision. Additionally, issues of accessibility, affordability, and equity must be addressed to ensure that psychedelic-assisted therapy is ethically and equitably available to those who may benefit from it.

Future Directions

The field of psychedelic research is rapidly evolving, with ongoing clinical trials and increased interest from the scientific community. Continued research is needed to strengthen the evidence base, refine protocols, and understand the long-term effects and potential risks of psychedelic-assisted therapy. Moreover, the integration of psychedelic treatments into mainstream mental health care requires collaboration between researchers, clinicians, policymakers, and regulatory bodies.

Conclusion

Research on the use of psychedelics in mental health treatment has shown promising results, suggesting their potential as a transformative approach in addressing various mental health conditions. While challenges and ethical considerations exist, ongoing research and collaboration have the potential to shape the future of mental health care and improve the well-being of individuals globally. The integration of psychedelics with traditional therapeutic approaches holds significant promise in expanding treatment options and providing novel interventions for individuals experiencing mental health challenges.

Ethical and Legal Considerations in Psychedelic-Assisted Therapy

Psychedelic-assisted therapy, a novel approach to mental health treatment, raises several important ethical and legal considerations. This section will explore these considerations, including the potential risks and benefits, the importance of informed consent, and the regulatory landscape surrounding psychedelic-assisted therapy.

Risks and Benefits

Like any medical intervention, psychedelic-assisted therapy carries both risks and potential benefits. Some of the risks associated with psychedelic use include psychological distress, anxiety, and adverse reactions. These risks may be amplified in individuals with pre-existing mental health conditions or those who are not adequately prepared for the experience. Additionally, the long-term effects and potential risks of repeated psychedelic use are still not fully understood.

On the other hand, psychedelic-assisted therapy has shown promising results in the treatment of various mental health disorders, including depression, post-traumatic stress disorder (PTSD), and substance use disorders. Studies have shown that psychedelic substances, such as psilocybin and MDMA, can enhance the therapeutic process by promoting emotional breakthroughs, facilitating the exploration of traumatic memories, and increasing feelings of connection and empathy. The potential benefits of psychedelic-assisted therapy extend beyond symptom reduction, with patients often reporting improved quality of life and increased well-being.

Informed Consent

Informed consent is a crucial ethical principle in medical treatment and research, and it holds particular significance in psychedelic-assisted therapy. Given the unique and potentially intense psychological experiences associated with psychedelics, ensuring that patients fully understand the risks, benefits, and potential outcomes is essential.

Informed consent in psychedelic-assisted therapy involves providing patients with accurate information about the treatment, including its purpose, procedures, potential risks, benefits, and alternative treatment options. It is also important to explain the nature of the psychedelic experience, emphasizing the potential for challenging or distressing aspects. This allows patients to make an autonomous and informed decision about whether to proceed with the therapy.

Moreover, practitioners must assess the psychological and physical suitability of individuals seeking psychedelic-assisted therapy. Screening protocols should be in place to identify individuals at risk of adverse reactions or those who may not derive significant benefits from the treatment. This helps ensure the safety and well-being of patients and prevents potential harm.

Regulatory Landscape

The legal and regulatory framework surrounding psychedelic-assisted therapy varies across different jurisdictions. In many countries, psychedelic substances are classified as Schedule I drugs, meaning they are deemed to have a high potential for abuse and no accepted medical use. As a result, their use in clinical settings is generally prohibited or heavily restricted.

However, there is a growing global movement advocating for the rescheduling of psychedelics to facilitate research and access to these therapies. In recent years, several countries and U.S. states have taken steps to decriminalize or legalize psychedelic substances, at least for medical or research purposes. These changes in policy reflect increasing recognition of the potential benefits of psychedelic-assisted therapy and the need to explore alternative treatment options for mental health disorders.

Ethics committees and regulatory bodies play a crucial role in ensuring the responsible and ethical use of psychedelics in therapeutic settings. They review research protocols, assess the qualifications and expertise of practitioners, and oversee the safety and well-being of patients. Additionally, ethical guidelines and professional standards are being developed to provide a framework for practitioners working in this emerging field.

Considerations for Future Development

As psychedelic-assisted therapy continues to evolve, it is essential to address certain considerations to safeguard patient well-being and optimize treatment outcomes. These considerations include:

- Training and Certification: Establishing standardized training programs and certification processes for practitioners to ensure competence, ethical practice, and adherence to safety protocols.

- Integration and Aftercare: Developing comprehensive integration and aftercare practices to support patients in processing their psychedelic experiences and integrating insights into their daily lives.

- Equity and Access: Ensuring that psychedelic-assisted therapy is accessible and affordable to diverse populations, preventing it from becoming an exclusive treatment option primarily available to privileged individuals.

- Long-Term Safety Monitoring: Conducting long-term follow-up studies to assess the potential risks and benefits of psychedelic-assisted therapy over extended periods and refine protocols accordingly.

- Public Education and Awareness: Raising public awareness about psychedelic-assisted therapy, dispelling misconceptions, and fostering an informed and supportive societal context for its use.

By addressing these considerations, the ethical and legal framework surrounding psychedelic-assisted therapy can continue to evolve in parallel with scientific advancements, ensuring the safe and responsible integration of these transformative treatments into mainstream mental health care.

In conclusion, ethical and legal considerations are paramount in psychedelic-assisted therapy. Balancing the potential risks and benefits, ensuring informed consent, and working within the evolving regulatory landscape are crucial for the safe and responsible use of psychedelics in therapeutic settings. Looking ahead, ongoing efforts to address these considerations will contribute to the ethical advancement of psychedelic-assisted therapy and its potential to revolutionize mental health care.

Epigenetics and Mental Health

Introduction to Epigenetics and Its Influence on Mental Health

In recent years, there has been growing interest in the field of epigenetics and its role in shaping our mental health. Epigenetics refers to the study of heritable changes in gene expression that occur without altering the underlying DNA sequence. It involves modifications to the structure of DNA or associated proteins, which can have profound effects on gene regulation and ultimately influence our physical and mental well-being.

Traditionally, the focus of mental health research has primarily been on genetic factors and environmental influences. However, the emerging field of epigenetics has enriched our understanding by highlighting the dynamic nature of gene expression and its susceptibility to modifications throughout our lifetime. Epigenetic mechanisms can be influenced by a variety of factors, including diet, stress, trauma, and environmental exposures, and can affect a wide range of mental health conditions, including depression, anxiety, addiction, and schizophrenia.

One of the key mechanisms through which epigenetic modifications occur is DNA methylation. This process involves the addition of a methyl group to specific regions of the DNA molecule, which can prevent the expression of certain genes. For example, studies have shown that increased DNA methylation of certain genes involved in stress response and emotional regulation is associated with a higher risk of developing mental health disorders.

Another important epigenetic mechanism is histone modification, which involves alterations to the proteins around which DNA is wound. These modifications can affect the accessibility of genes and impact their expression. Studies have shown that changes in histone acetylation, methylation, and phosphorylation can influence neural plasticity, synaptic function, and memory formation, all of which are critical for mental health.

Furthermore, recent research has also explored the role of non-coding RNAs, such as microRNAs, in epigenetic regulation. These small RNA molecules can bind to specific messenger RNAs and prevent their translation into proteins, thereby modulating gene expression. Dysregulation of microRNAs has been implicated in various mental health conditions, including depression and schizophrenia.

Understanding the influence of epigenetics on mental health has significant implications for developing personalized and targeted interventions. By identifying specific epigenetic markers associated with various disorders, researchers can potentially predict an individual's susceptibility to mental health conditions and tailor treatment strategies accordingly. Additionally, interventions targeting epigenetic mechanisms, such as dietary interventions or pharmacological agents, may provide new avenues for therapeutic intervention.

However, it is important to note that research in the field of epigenetics and mental health is still in its early stages, and many questions remain unanswered. The complexity of gene-environment interactions, the variability in epigenetic patterns across individuals, and the challenges of studying epigenetic changes in the brain are all factors that contribute to the current gaps in knowledge.

In conclusion, epigenetics opens up new perspectives on understanding the underlying mechanisms of mental health disorders. By exploring the influence of epigenetic modifications on gene expression, researchers can gain insights into the interactions between genetic and environmental factors. This knowledge holds great potential for the development of innovative therapeutic approaches, as well as advancing our understanding of mental health and well-being. However, further research is needed to fully elucidate the role of epigenetics in mental health and to translate these findings into clinical practice.

Key Concepts and Definitions

Epigenetics: The study of heritable changes in gene expression that occur without altering the underlying DNA sequence.

DNA Methylation: The addition of a methyl group to specific regions of the DNA molecule, which can prevent the expression of certain genes.

Histone Modification: Alterations to the proteins around which DNA is wound, which can affect the accessibility of genes and impact their expression.

Non-coding RNAs: RNA molecules that do not code for proteins but play a role in regulating gene expression. Examples include microRNAs.

Case Study: Epigenetics and Depression

To better understand the influence of epigenetics on mental health, let's consider a case study on depression. Depression is a complex mental health disorder influenced by a combination of genetic and environmental factors. Epigenetic modifications have been shown to play a role in the development and progression of depression.

Several studies have focused on DNA methylation patterns in individuals with depression. Researchers have identified specific genomic regions that show differential methylation between individuals with depression and those without. These regions are often associated with genes involved in neural development, stress response, and neurotransmitter signaling.

For instance, one study found that individuals with depression had increased DNA methylation at the promoter region of the serotonin transporter gene (SLC6A4), which is involved in the regulation of serotonin, a neurotransmitter implicated in mood regulation. This increased methylation was associated with reduced gene expression and impaired serotonin reuptake, potentially contributing to depressive symptoms.

Histone modifications have also been implicated in depression. Research has shown that alterations in histone acetylation and methylation patterns can affect the expression of genes involved in neuroplasticity and stress response. These changes may disrupt normal brain function and contribute to the development of depressive symptoms.

Furthermore, microRNAs have been identified as potential modifiers of gene expression in depression. Studies have found dysregulated microRNA levels in individuals with depression, suggesting their involvement in the regulation of genes related to mood and emotion.

This case study highlights the complex interplay between epigenetic modifications, genetic factors, and environmental influences in the development of depression. By understanding these epigenetic mechanisms, researchers can gain insights into the underlying biology of depression and potentially identify novel targets for therapeutic interventions.

Ethical Considerations in Epigenetics Research

The study of epigenetics raises important ethical considerations, particularly when it comes to mental health research. Some key ethical considerations include:

Informed Consent: Researchers must ensure that participants have a clear understanding of the potential risks and benefits of participating in epigenetics research. Informed consent should also address the potential implications of genetic and epigenetic information, particularly in the context of mental health.

Privacy and Confidentiality: Epigenetic research often involves the collection and analysis of sensitive genetic and personal information. Researchers must take steps to protect the privacy and confidentiality of participants, ensuring that data is securely stored and used only for research purposes.

Stigmatization and Discrimination: The discovery of epigenetic markers associated with mental health conditions raises concerns about stigmatization and discrimination. Ensuring that the disclosure of epigenetic information is done in a responsible and sensitive manner is crucial.

Equitable Access to Epigenetic Information: As epigenetic research advances, it is important to consider issues of equitable access to genetic and epigenetic information. Ensuring that individuals from diverse socio-economic backgrounds have access to the potential benefits of epigenetic research is essential.

Further Resources

Books

1. Meaney, M. J. (2019). Epigenetics and the biological definition of gene x environment interactions. Child development, 90(1), 4-13.

2. Champagne, F. A., & Curley, J. P. (2008). Epigenetic mechanisms mediating the long-term effects of maternal care on development. Neuroscience & Biobehavioral Reviews, 32(6), 1084-1096.

Articles

1. Weaver, I. C. G., Cervoni, N., Champagne, F. A., D'Alessio, A. C., Sharma, S., Seckl, J. R., ... & Meaney, M. J. (2004). Epigenetic programming by maternal behavior. Nature neuroscience, 7(8), 847-854.

2. Daskalakis, N. P., Bagot, R. C., Parker, K. J., Vinkers, C. H., & de Kloet, E. R. (2013).

3. The three‐generation Ketamine model in female rats: Disrupted experience‐dependent maturation of cortical parvalbumin interneurons. European Journal of Neuroscience, 37(5), 834-844.

Websites

1. The Epigenomics Program at the University of California, San Francisco: https://epigenomics.ucsf.edu/

2. National Institute of Mental Health: https://www.nimh.nih.gov/index.shtml

Summary

Epigenetics provides a novel perspective on the interplay between genetic and environmental factors in mental health. Understanding the mechanisms through which epigenetic modifications influence gene expression can shed light on the underlying biology of mental health disorders such as depression, anxiety, addiction, and schizophrenia. Epigenetic markers may also serve as potential targets for personalized therapies and interventions. However, further research is needed to fully explore the complex nature of epigenetic mechanisms and their implications for mental health. Ethical considerations surrounding the use of epigenetic information in research and clinical practice also deserve careful attention. Overall, epigenetics holds great promise for transforming our approach to mental health and well-being, paving the way for more effective and personalized treatments.

The Role of Environmental Factors on Gene Expression and Mental Wellness

Understanding the connection between environmental factors, gene expression, and mental wellness is crucial in unraveling the complexity of mental health disorders. This section explores the intricate interplay between our environment, our genes, and how they influence our mental well-being.

Environmental Factors and Gene Expression

Gene expression refers to the process by which information from a gene is used to create a functional product, such as a protein. Environmental factors can significantly influence gene expression, leading to changes in our biology and subsequent impacts on mental wellness. This concept is known as epigenetics.

Epigenetic modifications are reversible chemical alterations that can control gene expression without altering the underlying DNA sequence. One of the key mechanisms through which our environment can influence gene expression is through epigenetic modifications. These modifications can be influenced by various environmental factors, including our diet, stress levels, physical activity, exposure to toxins, and social interactions.

Nutrition and Gene Expression

Nutrition plays a vital role in determining our overall health, including our mental well-being. Emerging research suggests that specific nutrients can influence gene expression through epigenetic modifications, ultimately impacting mental wellness.

For example, omega-3 fatty acids found in fish oil have been associated with improved mental health outcomes, including reducing the risk of depression and anxiety disorders. These fatty acids can modulate gene expression involved in inflammation, synaptic plasticity, and neurotransmitter function, all of which are crucial for maintaining optimal mental wellness.

Similarly, the Mediterranean diet, rich in fruits, vegetables, whole grains, and healthy fats, has been linked to better mental health. Several components of this diet, such as antioxidants and polyphenols, can affect gene expression, leading to reduced inflammation and oxidative stress, which may help protect against mental health disorders.

Stress and Gene Expression

Chronic stress has been recognized as a significant risk factor for various mental health disorders. It is well-established that stress can affect gene expression patterns, particularly in brain regions involved in regulating emotions and stress responses.

Stress activates the hypothalamic-pituitary-adrenal (HPA) axis and triggers the release of stress hormones, such as cortisol. Prolonged exposure to elevated cortisol levels can lead to epigenetic modifications in genes related to stress regulation and neuronal function, increasing vulnerability to mental health conditions like anxiety, depression, and post-traumatic stress disorder (PTSD).

Understanding the mechanisms through which stress influences gene expression patterns can provide insights into developing targeted interventions for stress-related mental health disorders.

Toxins and Gene Expression

Exposure to environmental toxins can have detrimental effects on both physical and mental health. Certain toxins, such as heavy metals, pesticides, and air pollutants, have been shown to influence gene expression and contribute to the development or exacerbation of mental health disorders.

For example, exposure to lead has been linked to cognitive impairments and increased risk of attention-deficit/hyperactivity disorder (ADHD). Lead can affect the expression of genes involved in neurodevelopment and neurotransmitter systems, leading to altered brain functioning and increased susceptibility to mental health challenges.

Understanding how toxins interact with our genes and disrupt normal gene expression patterns is essential for developing strategies to mitigate their impact on mental wellness.

Social Interactions and Gene Expression

Our social environment can significantly influence gene expression patterns, shaping our mental well-being. Social support, relational experiences, and early-life interactions play crucial roles in gene regulation and mental wellness.

Positive social interactions and emotional support have been associated with reduced stress levels and improved mental health outcomes. Social support can modulate gene expression patterns related to stress responsiveness, inflammation, and immune functioning, promoting resilience and psychological well-being.

Conversely, social isolation and experiences of social adversity can contribute to detrimental gene expression patterns and increase the risk of mental health disorders. Chronic social stressors, such as bullying or social exclusion, can lead to epigenetic modifications in genes associated with stress regulation and emotional processing, predisposing individuals to mental health challenges.

Conclusion

The interplay between environmental factors and gene expression is a complex and dynamic process that significantly impacts mental wellness. Understanding how our environment influences gene expression patterns can provide valuable insights into the development, prevention, and treatment of mental health disorders.

By recognizing the role of environmental factors in shaping gene expression, we can identify modifiable factors that can be targeted for interventions and promote optimal mental well-being. This knowledge opens up new avenues for personalized approaches in mental health care, wherein interventions can be tailored to individuals based on their genetic and environmental profiles.

The field of epigenetics continues to advance our understanding of how environmental factors shape our gene expression, paving the way for innovative interventions and strategies to improve mental wellness. Further research, interdisciplinary collaborations, and continued exploration of the role of environmental factors in mental health are essential for shaping the future of mental health care.

Implications for Personalized Mental Health Treatment

Personalized mental health treatment is a rapidly evolving field that holds great potential for transforming the way we approach mental health care. By tailoring interventions to individual patients based on their unique characteristics, needs, and preferences, personalized treatment can improve the effectiveness and outcomes of mental health interventions. In this section, we will explore the implications of personalized mental health treatment and discuss how it can shape the future of mental health care.

Understanding Personalized Mental Health Treatment

Personalized mental health treatment involves customizing interventions to meet the specific needs of each individual. This approach recognizes that mental health disorders can vary widely from person to person, and there is no one-size-fits-all solution. By considering factors such as genetic makeup, biological markers, psychological traits, environmental influences, and cultural backgrounds, personalized treatment aims to provide targeted and effective interventions.

One of the key principles of personalized mental health treatment is the concept of precision medicine. This approach takes into account the heterogeneity of mental health disorders and focuses on identifying subtypes of disorders with distinct underlying mechanisms. By understanding the specific biological, genetic, and environmental factors that contribute to an individual's mental health condition, treatment can be tailored to address these factors and improve outcomes.

Advancements in Personalized Mental Health Treatment

Advancements in technologies, research methodologies, and understanding of mental health disorders have paved the way for personalized treatment approaches. Here are some key advancements with implications for personalized mental health treatment:

Genomics and Biomarkers: The field of genomics has provided valuable insights into the genetic basis of mental health disorders. By identifying specific genetic variations associated with different disorders, researchers can develop targeted interventions based on an individual's genetic profile. Biomarkers, such as neuroimaging or blood-based markers, can also provide objective measures of treatment response and help guide personalized interventions.

Machine Learning and Predictive Analytics: Machine learning algorithms can analyze large datasets and identify patterns and predictors of treatment response. By leveraging these techniques, clinicians can make more accurate predictions about a patient's prognosis and tailor treatments accordingly. For example, machine learning can help identify which individuals are likely to benefit from a specific medication or therapy approach.

Digital Mental Health Tools: Advancements in technology have given rise to digital mental health tools, such as smartphone apps and wearable devices, that can collect real-time data on individuals' mental health. These tools can provide valuable information about an individual's symptoms, behaviors, and treatment response, allowing for personalized interventions that are continuously adapted and optimized.

Challenges and Considerations

While personalized mental health treatment shows great promise, it also presents challenges and considerations that need to be addressed:

Ethical and Privacy Concerns: The use of genetic information, biomarkers, and digital health data raises ethical and privacy concerns. It is crucial to ensure that individuals' privacy is protected, and their data is used responsibly and with informed consent. Additionally, careful consideration must be given to issues of equity and access, as personalized treatments may not be accessible or affordable for everyone.

Integration into Clinical Practice: Integrating personalized mental health treatment into clinical practice poses challenges in terms of training, resources, and infrastructure. Clinicians need to be equipped with the knowledge and skills to implement personalized approaches effectively. Health systems must also provide the necessary support and resources to implement personalized treatments on a larger scale.

Evidence and Research: As personalized mental health treatment is a relatively new field, more research is needed to establish its efficacy and effectiveness. Rigorous studies are needed to evaluate the impact of personalized interventions on treatment outcomes, cost-effectiveness, and long-term benefits. Collaborative efforts between researchers, clinicians, and policymakers are essential to generating robust evidence and driving the adoption of personalized treatments.

Case Study: Applying Personalized Treatment for Depression

To illustrate the implications of personalized mental health treatment, let's consider a case study of depression. Traditional treatment approaches for depression often involve a combination of medication and psychotherapy. However, response rates to these interventions can vary significantly among individuals. With personalized treatment, the focus shifts to identifying the underlying causes and tailoring interventions accordingly.

For instance, a personalized approach might consider factors such as the individual's genetic predisposition, neurotransmitter imbalances, psychosocial stressors, and lifestyle factors. Genetic testing can reveal variations in genes associated with treatment response, helping guide medication selection. Neuroimaging techniques can identify brain regions implicated in an individual's depression, leading to targeted interventions such as transcranial magnetic stimulation.

Furthermore, personalized treatment may involve addressing psychosocial factors such as trauma history, social support networks, and lifestyle choices. Cognitive-behavioral therapy (CBT) can be adapted to target specific cognitive distortions or maladaptive coping strategies identified in an individual's case. Lifestyle modifications, including exercise, nutrition, and sleep improvements, can also be integrated into the treatment plan based on the individual's needs and preferences.

By tailoring interventions based on these personalized factors, the likelihood of achieving positive treatment outcomes may increase. The individual's active involvement and collaboration in the treatment process can also enhance engagement and adherence to the personalized interventions.

Conclusion

Personalized mental health treatment holds significant promise for improving the effectiveness and outcomes of mental health interventions. By considering individual characteristics, needs, and preferences, personalized approaches can optimize treatment selection and delivery. However, the successful implementation of personalized treatment requires addressing ethical, practical, and research challenges. Ongoing research, collaboration, and a strong commitment to ensuring equitable access to personalized interventions are key to realizing the full potential of personalized mental health treatment.

Cultural Considerations in Mental Health Research

Cultural Competence in Mental Health Care

Cultural competence plays a crucial role in providing effective mental health care to diverse populations. It involves understanding and respecting the cultural beliefs, values, and practices that influence an individual's perception of mental health and well-being. By incorporating cultural competence into mental health care, clinicians can better address the unique needs and challenges faced by individuals from different cultural backgrounds. In this section, we will explore the importance of cultural competence, strategies for developing cultural competence in mental health care, and the benefits of integrating cultural perspectives in treatment.

Understanding Cultural Competence

Cultural competence is the ability to understand and effectively respond to the cultural and linguistic needs of individuals from diverse backgrounds. It requires clinicians to be aware of their own biases and assumptions, and to approach each patient with an open mind. Cultural competence is not a one-size-fits-all approach; instead, it recognizes the importance of tailoring treatment plans to meet the specific needs and values of each individual.

In mental health care, cultural competence is essential because culture influences how individuals perceive and express mental health concerns, seek help, and engage in treatment. By understanding cultural factors, clinicians can develop a deeper understanding of their patients' experiences, increase treatment adherence, and enhance overall treatment outcomes.

Strategies for Developing Cultural Competence

Developing cultural competence is a continuous process that requires self-reflection, education, and open-mindedness. Here are some strategies to enhance cultural competence in mental health care:

1. Self-awareness: Clinicians must first recognize their own cultural biases and assumptions. They can engage in activities such as self-reflection, attending cultural humility workshops, or participating in intercultural experiences to increase their self-awareness.

2. Cultural humility: Cultivating a mindset of cultural humility involves recognizing that no single person can fully understand the complexities of another person's culture. Clinicians should approach each patient with humility, curiosity, and a willingness to learn from and about their culture.

3. Education and training: Clinicians should actively pursue education and training opportunities to learn about the cultures they serve. This can include attending cultural competency workshops, participating in diversity and inclusion training, or seeking mentorship from colleagues with expertise in specific cultural groups.

4. Collaboration and consultation: Clinicians should be open to seeking collaboration and consultation with individuals from the communities they serve. This collaboration can help bridge gaps in knowledge and understanding and ensure culturally appropriate care.

5. Flexibility in treatment approaches: Recognizing that different cultures may have distinct beliefs and practices regarding mental health, clinicians should be flexible in adapting treatment approaches to align with the patient's cultural

context. This may involve incorporating traditional healing practices, involving family members in treatment, or modifying treatment modalities.

Benefits of Integrating Cultural Perspectives

Integrating cultural perspectives in mental health care has several benefits:

1. Improved engagement and treatment adherence: When clinicians acknowledge and respect the patient's cultural values and beliefs, they are more likely to build trust and establish a therapeutic alliance. This can lead to increased engagement in treatment and improved treatment adherence.

2. Enhanced accuracy and effectiveness of assessment: By understanding how culture shapes individuals' experiences and expression of mental health symptoms, clinicians can conduct more accurate and culturally sensitive assessments. This can lead to more appropriate diagnoses and treatment plans.

3. Increased patient satisfaction and trust: When patients feel that their cultural backgrounds are understood and respected, they are more likely to feel satisfied with their care and trust their clinicians. This can contribute to positive treatment outcomes and patient well-being.

4. Reduction in disparities: Cultural competence can help address mental health disparities experienced by marginalized communities. By understanding the unique challenges faced by different cultural groups, clinicians can develop targeted interventions and advocate for equitable access to mental health care.

5. Promotion of cultural resilience and strengths: Cultural competence acknowledges the resilience, strengths, and resources within a cultural group. By integrating cultural perspectives, clinicians can promote cultural strengths, empower individuals, and foster positive mental health outcomes.

In summary, cultural competence is critical in providing effective mental health care. By understanding and incorporating cultural perspectives, clinicians can build trust, tailor treatment plans to meet individual needs, and address mental health disparities. Developing cultural competence requires self-awareness, education, and collaboration. By embracing cultural competence, clinicians can contribute to more inclusive and effective mental health care practices.

Intersectionality and Mental Health

Intersectionality is a concept that recognizes the interconnected nature of various social identities and the ways in which they intersect to shape an individual's experiences and disadvantages in society. It emphasizes that individuals possess multiple dimensions of identity, such as race, gender, sexuality, socio-economic status, and disability, that interact and influence their lived experiences.

In the context of mental health, intersectionality provides a framework to understand how various social identities can intersect and contribute to unique experiences and challenges in relation to mental well-being. It recognizes that mental health is not solely determined by individual factors but is significantly influenced by broader social and structural factors.

Understanding the Intersections of Identity and Mental Health

Intersectionality helps us understand that individuals with multiple marginalized identities may face unique mental health challenges resulting from the shared effects of multiple forms of discrimination and oppression. For example, a queer person of color may experience stress and stigma related to both their racial and sexual identity, which can impact their mental health.

Moreover, intersectionality also acknowledges that individuals who possess privileged identities in some aspects of their lives may still experience mental health difficulties due to other intersecting dimensions of their identity. This recognition underscores the importance of examining mental health through an intersectional lens, as it allows for a nuanced understanding of the experiences of different individuals.

The Impact of Intersectionality on Mental Health Disparities

The application of an intersectional perspective in mental health research highlights the existence of significant disparities in mental health outcomes across different social groups. For instance, studies have shown that individuals who identify as Black, Indigenous, and People of Color (BIPOC), as well as individuals who identify as LGBTQ+, are at a higher risk of experiencing mental health issues compared to their white and heterosexual counterparts.

These disparities can be attributed to various intersecting factors, including societal discrimination, systemic inequalities, cultural differences in help-seeking behaviors, and limited access to culturally responsive mental health services. By recognizing these intersections, mental health practitioners can develop more effective strategies and interventions to address the mental health disparities experienced by marginalized communities.

Practices for Culturally Competent Mental Health Support

To effectively address the mental health needs of individuals from diverse backgrounds, mental health professionals must adopt culturally competent practices. Culturally competent care acknowledges and respects the influence of cultural, social, and historical factors on mental health and ensures that mental health services are sensitive to and inclusive of diverse experiences.

Some key practices for providing culturally competent mental health support include:

- **Cultural awareness and self-reflection:** Mental health professionals should continuously examine their own biases and assumptions regarding different social identities and actively engage in self-reflection to develop cultural humility.

- **Intersectional assessment:** When conducting assessments, mental health practitioners should take a comprehensive approach that considers the intersectional identities and experiences of individuals and how they may impact their mental health.

- **Collaborative care:** Collaborating with clients to develop treatment plans that consider their unique socio-cultural needs and preferences promotes trust and engagement in the therapeutic process.

- **Culturally responsive interventions:** Tailoring interventions to be congruent with clients' cultural values, beliefs, and practices helps ensure that mental health support is relevant and effective.

- **Community engagement and advocacy:** Mental health professionals should actively engage with communities and advocate for inclusive policies and practices that address the intersecting needs of marginalized individuals.

By integrating these practices into mental health care, professionals can better address the diverse needs and experiences of individuals from different intersecting identities.

Case Study: Intersectionality and Mental Health in the LGBTQ+ Community

An example that highlights the importance of intersectionality in mental health is the experiences of individuals within the LGBTQ+ community. LGBTQ+

individuals can face unique mental health challenges due to the intersection of their sexual orientation, gender identity, and other factors such as race and socio-economic status.

Studies have shown that LGBTQ+ individuals are at a higher risk of experiencing mental health disorders, such as depression, anxiety, and substance abuse, compared to the general population. This increased risk can be attributed to multiple intersecting factors, including the stigma and discrimination faced by LGBTQ+ individuals, the lack of social support networks, and barriers to accessing affirming mental health care.

To address these intersecting challenges, mental health practitioners need to provide LGBTQ+ individuals with culturally competent care that acknowledges and affirms their particularities. This can include creating safe and inclusive spaces, understanding the unique mental health needs of different LGBTQ+ subgroups, and incorporating LGBTQ+-affirming approaches in therapy.

Call to Action

Recognizing and addressing intersectionality in mental health research, policy, and practice is essential for promoting equity and social justice in mental health care. It is crucial to address the unique experiences and challenges faced by individuals with intersecting identities to ensure that mental health support is inclusive and effective for all.

To accomplish this, it is necessary to integrate intersectionality into mental health education and training programs for mental health professionals, increase the representation of diverse voices and experiences in research, and advocate for policies that address the intersecting needs of marginalized populations.

By embracing an intersectional approach in mental health, we can strive towards a more equitable, inclusive, and holistic mental health care system where everyone's mental well-being is valued and supported.

Incorporating Cultural Perspectives in Research Design and Intervention Development

When conducting research and developing interventions in the field of mental health, it is crucial to recognize and incorporate cultural perspectives. Culture plays a significant role in shaping individuals' beliefs, attitudes, and behaviors related to mental health and well-being. By understanding the cultural context, researchers and practitioners can develop more effective and culturally sensitive approaches to address mental health concerns.

Understanding Culture and its Impact on Mental Health

Culture refers to the beliefs, values, practices, and behaviors shared by a specific group of people. It encompasses various aspects such as ethnicity, race, socioeconomic status, religion, language, and gender, among others. These cultural factors influence how individuals perceive and experience mental health issues.

For example, in some cultures, mental health problems may be stigmatized or seen as a sign of weakness. This stigma can prevent individuals from seeking help and may impact their overall well-being. Additionally, cultural norms and values shape the types of treatments and interventions that individuals find acceptable or effective.

Cultural Competence in Research Design

Incorporating cultural perspectives into research design is essential to ensure that studies are relevant and meaningful for diverse populations. Cultural competence involves respecting and considering cultural differences in study design, data collection, and analysis. Here are some key considerations for incorporating cultural perspectives in research:

1. **Forming diverse research teams:** Researchers from different cultural backgrounds should collaborate to bring their unique perspectives and insights. This diversity enhances the validity and cultural sensitivity of the research.

2. **Culturally appropriate measures:** Researchers should use validated measures that are culturally appropriate and relevant to the population being studied. This ensures that the instruments capture the nuances of cultural experiences and beliefs.

3. **Language and literacy considerations:** Language barriers and low literacy levels can affect the accuracy of data collection. Researchers should provide materials in the participants' preferred language and ensure that they are easily understandable.

4. **Sampling strategies:** Researchers should strive for diverse and representative samples that include individuals from different cultural backgrounds. This helps to capture the full range of experiences and perspectives within a given cultural group.

Intervention Development with Cultural Sensitivity

Developing culturally sensitive interventions requires an understanding of the cultural context, beliefs, and preferences of the target population. These interventions should respect cultural values, be accessible, and address the unique challenges faced by different cultural groups. Here are some considerations for developing culturally sensitive interventions:

1. **Cultural adaptation:** Interventions should be adapted to fit the cultural beliefs, practices, and values of the target population. This may involve modifying content, language, or delivery methods to ensure they align with cultural norms.

2. **Collaboration with community stakeholders:** Engaging with community leaders, organizations, and individuals with expertise in the cultural group being targeted can provide valuable insights and ensure the intervention's relevance.

3. **Incorporating traditional healing practices:** Many cultures have traditional healing practices that can complement conventional mental health treatments. Integrating these practices into interventions can enhance acceptability and effectiveness.

4. **Training culturally competent practitioners:** Ensuring that practitioners delivering the interventions are culturally competent is essential. They should have an understanding and appreciation of the cultural beliefs and practices of the individuals they serve.

Ethical Considerations

When incorporating cultural perspectives in research and intervention development, ethical considerations are paramount. Researchers and practitioners must navigate potential ethical challenges to ensure the well-being and autonomy of participants. Here are some ethical considerations:

1. **Informed consent:** Researchers must ensure that participants fully understand the purpose, risks, and benefits of participating in the study. This includes ensuring cultural appropriateness in obtaining informed consent.

2. **Confidentiality and privacy:** Respecting cultural norms around confidentiality and privacy is important. Researchers should establish appropriate safeguards for protecting participants' personal and cultural identity.

3. **Power dynamics:** Researchers must be mindful of power imbalances between themselves and the research participants, especially when working with marginalized cultural groups. Ensuring equitable partnerships and involving participants in decision-making processes can help mitigate these imbalances.

Case Example: Cultural Perspectives in Mental Health Research

To illustrate the importance of incorporating cultural perspectives, let's consider a case example involving depression research in a multicultural society. Researchers aiming to study the effectiveness of CBT-based interventions for depression would need to consider the following:

1. **Language and cultural relevance:** The researchers should ensure that the intervention materials and assessments are available in different languages spoken by the diverse population to facilitate participation and accurate data collection.

2. **Cultural idioms of distress:** Understanding cultural expressions of distress is crucial. For instance, some cultural groups may not use the term "depression" but may describe emotional distress in other ways. Researchers should be sensitive to these cultural idioms of distress when assessing and discussing mental health symptoms.

3. **Help-seeking behaviors:** Cultural attitudes towards seeking help for mental health issues can influence the recruitment and retention of participants. Researchers should carefully consider these attitudes to develop effective recruitment strategies.

4. **Culturally responsive interventions:** The researchers should consider adapting the CBT intervention to incorporate cultural values, beliefs, and practices. This could involve tailoring examples and case studies to be more culturally relevant and acceptable for the target population.

By incorporating these cultural perspectives, the research can yield more accurate and applicable results, providing valuable insights into the effectiveness of CBT-based interventions for depression in the multicultural society under study.

Conclusion

Incorporating cultural perspectives in research design and intervention development is essential to ensure that mental health studies are relevant, respectful, and effective. By recognizing and addressing the cultural nuances, researchers and practitioners can develop interventions that are sensitive to diverse populations, resulting in better mental health outcomes. Embracing cultural diversity and fostering collaboration will help shape a more inclusive and transformative mental health landscape.

The Future of Mental Health and Wellbeing

Challenges and Opportunities for Mental Health Care

Access and Equity in Mental Health Services

Access and equity in mental health services are crucial factors in ensuring that individuals receive the care they need regardless of their background or circumstances. In many societies, there are significant disparities in access to mental health services, with certain populations facing barriers that prevent them from receiving adequate care. In this section, we will explore the challenges related to access and equity in mental health services and discuss strategies to address these issues.

Understanding Access to Mental Health Services

Access to mental health services refers to the ease with which individuals can obtain the necessary care and support for their mental health concerns. It encompasses several dimensions, including availability, affordability, acceptability, and appropriateness of services. Unfortunately, many individuals face significant barriers that hinder their access to mental health care.

    1. **Geographical Barriers:** One common challenge is the lack of mental health care services in certain areas, especially in rural or remote regions. Limited availability of mental health professionals and facilities can make it difficult for individuals in these areas to access timely and appropriate care.

    2. **Financial Barriers:** The cost of mental health services can be a significant barrier for many individuals, particularly those without insurance coverage or with limited financial resources. High out-of-pocket expenses for treatment and medication can deter individuals from seeking or continuing mental health care.

3. **Cultural and Linguistic Barriers:** Sociocultural factors can also create barriers to accessing mental health services. Language barriers, cultural stigma, and lack of culturally competent care can deter individuals from seeking help. Moreover, individuals from marginalized communities may face discrimination, which further exacerbates their vulnerability and limits their access to appropriate care.

4. **Systemic Barriers:** The structure and organization of mental health care systems can also present obstacles to access and equity. Long waiting times, limited appointment availability, and fragmented care coordination can impede individuals' ability to receive continuous and comprehensive care.

Addressing Barriers to Access in Mental Health Services

Addressing barriers to access and promoting equity in mental health services requires a multi-faceted approach that involves stakeholders at various levels. Here, we will discuss strategies to address the challenges and improve access to mental health care for all individuals.

1. **Improving Service Availability:** One priority is to expand the availability of mental health services, particularly in underserved areas. This can be achieved by increasing the number of trained mental health professionals, improving infrastructure, and establishing telehealth or mobile clinics to reach individuals in remote areas.

2. **Enhancing Affordability:** To improve affordability, it is essential to advocate for mental health parity, which ensures that mental health services are covered by insurance plans at the same level as physical health services. Additionally, increasing funding for mental health programs and subsidizing costs for low-income individuals can reduce financial barriers.

3. **Promoting Cultural Competence:** Mental health services should be culturally sensitive and responsive to the needs of diverse populations. This can be achieved by providing cultural competence training to mental health professionals, recruiting diverse staff, and incorporating cultural perspectives into treatment approaches.

4. **Improving Care Coordination:** Streamlining care coordination can enhance access to mental health services. This can involve implementing referral networks, integrating mental health care with primary care services, and utilizing electronic health records to improve communication and continuity of care.

5. **Implementing Outreach and Awareness Programs:** Outreach programs can play a crucial role in reaching individuals who may be unaware of available mental health services or hesitant to seek help. These programs should focus on increasing

mental health literacy, reducing stigma, and educating communities about available resources.

6. **Advocacy and Policy Development**: Advocacy efforts are essential for creating lasting change in mental health care systems. It involves raising awareness, influencing policies, and advocating for increased funding and resources for mental health services. By working collaboratively with policymakers, advocacy groups can help shape policies that promote access and equity.

Real-World Example

To illustrate the importance of addressing access and equity, let us consider a real-world example:

In a rural community, there is a lack of mental health services, and individuals with mental health concerns often have to travel long distances to access the nearest mental health professional. The financial burden of transportation, coupled with the limited availability of services, prevents many individuals from seeking treatment.

To address this issue, a community-based organization collaborates with local health authorities to establish a telehealth program. Through this program, individuals can receive mental health consultations and therapy sessions remotely, eliminating the need for travel. The program also offers financial assistance to cover the cost of telehealth services for low-income individuals. Additionally, the organization conducts community outreach to raise awareness about mental health and the availability of remote services.

By implementing this telehealth program, the community improves access to mental health care, particularly for those who face geographical and financial barriers. This initiative not only addresses access and equity concerns but also promotes early intervention and supports individuals in maintaining their mental wellbeing.

Conclusion

Ensuring access and equity in mental health services is essential for promoting the overall wellbeing of individuals and communities. By recognizing and addressing the barriers that limit access to care, we can work towards a more inclusive and equitable mental health care system. Through collaboration, advocacy, and the implementation of targeted strategies, we can make significant strides in improving access and fostering equity in mental health services.

Addressing Socioeconomic and Structural Influences on Mental Health

Socioeconomic and structural influences play a significant role in shaping mental health outcomes. These influences can create barriers to accessing mental health services, exacerbate mental health disparities, and contribute to the development and persistence of mental health conditions. In this section, we will explore the impact of socioeconomic and structural factors on mental health and discuss strategies for addressing these influences.

The Impact of Socioeconomic Factors on Mental Health

Socioeconomic factors, such as income, education, employment, and social status, significantly influence mental health outcomes. Research has consistently shown that individuals from lower socioeconomic backgrounds are at an increased risk of mental health disorders compared to those with higher socioeconomic status.

Financial stress, unstable employment, and inadequate access to resources like housing and healthcare can create chronic stress, increasing the risk of mental health problems. Additionally, limited educational opportunities and social support networks can further contribute to mental health disparities.

To address these socioeconomic influences, it is essential to implement policies that promote economic stability, reduce income inequality, and provide equal opportunities for education and employment. Investing in social welfare programs, affordable housing, and job training can help alleviate the financial burdens that contribute to mental health problems.

Structural Influences on Mental Health

Structural factors refer to the social, political, and environmental conditions that shape mental health outcomes. These factors include discrimination, social exclusion, urbanization, and environmental hazards. Structural influences can have a profound impact on mental health by creating conditions that perpetuate inequality and marginalization.

Discrimination based on race, ethnicity, gender, sexuality, or disability can lead to significant psychological distress and increase the risk of mental health disorders. Social exclusion, such as isolation or exclusion from community resources, can also have detrimental effects on mental wellbeing.

Urbanization and the built environment play a role in mental health outcomes. Urban areas with limited access to green spaces, high levels of noise, and pollution have been associated with higher rates of mental health problems.

Addressing structural influences on mental health requires a holistic approach that involves policy changes, community engagement, and advocacy. Efforts should focus on combating discrimination, promoting inclusivity, and creating environments that support mental wellbeing. This can include implementing anti-discrimination policies, increasing access to resources in marginalized communities, and designing cities and neighborhoods that prioritize mental health.

Integrating Socioeconomic and Structural Approaches

To effectively address socioeconomic and structural influences on mental health, it is crucial to integrate these approaches into mental health practices and policies. This integration requires collaboration between mental health professionals, policymakers, community organizations, and individuals with lived experiences of mental health challenges.

Mental health services need to be made accessible and affordable to individuals from all socioeconomic backgrounds. This can involve implementing sliding-scale fee structures, increasing the availability of mental health services in underserved areas, and integrating mental health support into primary care settings.

Additionally, mental health practitioners should receive training on cultural competency and trauma-informed care to better understand and address the specific needs of individuals from diverse socioeconomic backgrounds. By understanding the intersectionality of socioeconomic and structural influences on mental health, practitioners can develop tailored interventions and support systems.

Building partnerships with community organizations can also help address socioeconomic and structural influences on mental health. Collaborating with local agencies and grassroots initiatives can create opportunities for community engagement, resource-sharing, and advocacy. These partnerships can help address not only individual mental health needs but also broader systemic issues.

Conclusion

Addressing socioeconomic and structural influences on mental health is crucial for ensuring equitable access to quality mental health care and reducing mental health disparities. By implementing policies that promote economic stability, combat discrimination, and create supportive environments, we can create a transformed mental health landscape that promotes the wellbeing of all individuals, regardless of their socioeconomic backgrounds.

It is imperative that we continue to research and advocate for the integration of socioeconomic and structural approaches in mental health care, as this is vital to improving outcomes for individuals and communities. By acknowledging and addressing these influences, we can work towards a future where mental health resources and support are accessible to all.

Integrating Mental Health into Primary Care Settings

Integrating mental health into primary care settings is a crucial step towards improving access to mental health services and achieving better overall health outcomes for individuals. Primary care providers play a key role in identifying and addressing mental health concerns, as they are often the first point of contact for patients seeking healthcare. This section will explore the importance of integrating mental health into primary care, the challenges faced in doing so, and potential strategies for successful integration.

The Importance of Integrated Care

Mental health disorders are prevalent worldwide, with estimates suggesting that approximately 1 in 4 individuals will experience a mental health issue at some point in their lives. Despite the high prevalence, mental health disorders often go undiagnosed and untreated. This can lead to significant negative impacts on individuals' quality of life, as well as increased healthcare costs. Integrated care, which combines physical and mental health services, has been shown to be effective in improving outcomes for patients with mental health issues.

One of the key benefits of integrating mental health into primary care is improved access to care. By embedding mental health services within primary care settings, individuals can receive timely and convenient treatment without the need for additional referrals. This is particularly important for individuals who may face barriers to accessing specialized mental health services, such as limited financial resources, long wait times, or stigma associated with seeking mental health treatment.

Integrating mental health into primary care also helps address the issue of fragmentation in healthcare. Mental health and physical health are interconnected, and it is essential to recognize and address the holistic needs of individuals. By offering comprehensive care that considers the physical, mental, and social aspects of health, integrated care promotes a more holistic and patient-centered approach.

Challenges in Integration

Despite the benefits, there are several challenges in integrating mental health into primary care settings. These challenges stem from various factors, including limited resources, inadequate training, and persistent stigma surrounding mental health.

One major challenge is the shortage of mental health professionals. The demand for mental health services often exceeds the supply of qualified professionals, particularly in underserved areas. This shortage can limit the extent to which mental health services can be fully integrated into primary care settings. Collaborative models, such as telehealth and consultations with psychiatric specialists, can help bridge this gap and ensure patients receive the appropriate care.

Another challenge is the need for enhanced training for primary care providers. While primary care providers are skilled in addressing physical health concerns, they may lack the specialized training required to diagnose and manage mental health conditions. Integrating mental health into primary care necessitates ongoing training and support for primary care providers to enhance their knowledge and skills in mental health assessment, treatment, and referral.

Stigma surrounding mental health remains a significant barrier to integration. Many individuals still face discrimination and judgment when seeking mental health support, which can deter them from disclosing their concerns to primary care providers. Addressing stigma requires a multifaceted approach, including public education campaigns, community outreach, and the fostering of a non-judgmental and supportive environment within primary care settings.

Strategies for Integration

Successfully integrating mental health into primary care requires a comprehensive approach that addresses the challenges discussed earlier. Here are some strategies to facilitate integration:

1. Collaborative care models: Implementing collaborative care models, such as the Collaborative Care Model, can enhance coordination among primary care providers, mental health specialists, and other healthcare professionals. This model involves regular communication and shared decision-making to ensure patients receive integrated care.

2. Training and education: Investment in training and education programs for primary care providers is essential. These programs should focus on enhancing mental health literacy, improving diagnostic skills, providing evidence-based treatment approaches, and offering ongoing support and consultation.

3. Screening and assessment tools: Integrating systematic screening and assessment tools within primary care settings can help identify individuals with mental health concerns early on. Various validated screening tools, such as the Patient Health Questionnaire (PHQ-9) for depression and the Generalized Anxiety Disorder (GAD-7) questionnaire, can be used to facilitate screening.

4. Care coordination and referral networks: Establishing strong referral networks and care coordination systems between primary care providers and mental health specialists is crucial. Clear pathways for referrals, timely communication, and shared care plans can ensure seamless transitions and continuity of care for patients.

5. Patient empowerment and education: Empowering patients through mental health education, self-help resources, and shared decision-making can promote active engagement in their care. Providing information about available mental health services, treatment options, and self-management strategies can support patients in making informed decisions and taking an active role in their mental health.

6. Addressing health system barriers: Advocacy efforts should be directed towards addressing systemic barriers, such as reimbursement challenges, policy gaps, and resource allocation. Policy changes and financial incentives can incentivize the integration of mental health services into primary care settings.

Overall, integrating mental health into primary care settings requires a collaborative and multidimensional approach. By addressing the challenges and implementing effective strategies, the delivery of comprehensive care that considers both physical and mental health can be achieved, leading to improved outcomes for individuals and their communities.

Conclusion

Integrating mental health into primary care settings is paramount to address the growing burden of mental health disorders and improve overall health outcomes. The benefits of integrated care, such as improved access, holistic care, and better coordination, make it an essential component of modern healthcare systems.

While challenges exist, including resource constraints, training needs, and stigma, implementing strategies like collaborative care models, enhanced training, systematic screening, and care coordination can help overcome these barriers. Additionally, empowering patients through education and involvement in decision-making processes, as well as advocating for policy changes and addressing systemic barriers, are crucial steps towards successful integration.

The future of mental health care lies in the convergence of physical and mental health services, recognizing and addressing the interconnectedness of these domains. By embracing integration, healthcare systems can shape a transformed mental health landscape, promoting well-being and improving the lives of individuals and communities worldwide.

Resources for Further Reading

1. World Health Organization. (2008). Integrating mental health into primary care: a global perspective. Retrieved from https://www.who.int/mental_health/resources/mentalhealth_PHC_2008.pdf

2. Gilbody, S., Bower, P., Fletcher, J., Richards, D., & Sutton, A. J. (2006). Collaborative care for depression: a cumulative meta-analysis and review of longer-term outcomes. Archives of Internal Medicine, 166(21), 2314-2321.

3. Søgaard, A. J., Selmer, R., Bjertness, E., Thelle, D., & Nafstad, P. (2004). Cohort profile: The Oslo Health Study (HUBRO). International Journal of Epidemiology, 35(5), 1143-1147.

4. Mental Health America. (n.d.). Integrated care. Retrieved from https://www.mhanational.org/issues/integrated-care

5. Substance Abuse and Mental Health Services Administration. (2018). Primary and behavioral health care integration (PBHCI) program. Retrieved from https://www.samhsa.gov/sites/default/files/pbhci_report.pdf

Emerging Trends in Mental Health Research and Practice

Personalized Medicine in Mental Health

Personalized medicine is an emerging field that aims to tailor medical treatments to individual patients, taking into account their unique genetic makeup, lifestyle factors, and other personal characteristics. This approach recognizes that there is no "one-size-fits-all" solution when it comes to healthcare, including mental health. In recent years, personalized medicine has gained momentum in various medical specialties, and its principles are now being applied to mental health care as well.

Understanding Personalized Medicine

Personalized medicine in mental health is based on the concept that effective treatment should consider an individual's specific biological, psychological, and social factors, rather than relying solely on generalized treatment protocols. It recognizes that mental health disorders are complex and can vary widely between individuals, and that factors such as genetic predisposition, environmental influences, and lifestyle choices can all play a role in the development and progression of these disorders.

The goal of personalized medicine in mental health is to improve treatment outcomes by tailoring interventions to the unique needs of each individual. This approach takes into account various factors, including genetic variations, biomarkers, response to previous treatments, and personal preferences, to develop a treatment plan that is most likely to be effective for a specific individual.

Integration of Genomics and Mental Health

One of the key components of personalized medicine in mental health is the integration of genomics. Genomics is the study of an individual's genetic material, including their DNA sequence and variations in genes. By analyzing an individual's genetic profile, researchers can gain insights into their susceptibility to certain mental health disorders, their responsiveness to specific medications, and their risk of adverse drug reactions.

The field of psychiatric genetics has made significant strides in recent years, identifying various genetic variants that are associated with an increased risk of mental health disorders. For example, specific gene variations have been linked to an increased risk of developing conditions such as schizophrenia, bipolar disorder, and major depressive disorder. By identifying these genetic markers, clinicians can potentially predict an individual's susceptibility to these disorders and develop targeted intervention strategies.

Pharmacogenomics in Mental Health

Pharmacogenomics is a branch of personalized medicine that focuses on how an individual's genetic makeup affects their response to medications. In mental health care, pharmacogenomic testing can provide insights into an individual's likelihood of responding to a particular medication, as well as their risk of experiencing adverse drug reactions or side effects.

By analyzing an individual's genetic profile, clinicians can identify genetic variations that impact the metabolism, efficacy, and safety of psychiatric medications. This information can guide treatment decisions, helping clinicians to select medications that are more likely to be effective and well-tolerated by the patient.

For example, some individuals may have variations in genes that affect how their bodies metabolize certain medications. This can result in higher or lower blood levels of the medication, potentially leading to treatment failure or increased risk of side effects. By considering these genetic variations, clinicians can personalize medication dosages and select alternative medications with a higher likelihood of success.

Challenges and Limitations

While personalized medicine holds great promise for the field of mental health care, there are also challenges and limitations that need to be addressed.

One of the primary challenges is the complexity of mental health disorders themselves. Unlike some other medical conditions, mental health disorders often involve a combination of biological, psychological, and social factors. Understanding how these different factors interact and contribute to a person's symptoms can be challenging, and it may take time and further research to develop comprehensive personalized treatment approaches.

Another challenge is the availability and accessibility of genetic testing and other personalized medicine tools. Although genetic testing has become more widely available in recent years, it is not yet a routine part of mental health care in many settings. Cost, insurance coverage, and privacy concerns are some of the barriers that need to be addressed to ensure equal access to personalized medicine approaches.

Furthermore, it is essential to recognize that personalized medicine is not a panacea. While it can improve treatment outcomes for many individuals, it is not a guarantee of success. Mental health disorders are highly complex and multifaceted, and personalized medicine approaches should always be considered as part of a comprehensive treatment plan that includes psychotherapy, lifestyle interventions, and support from healthcare professionals.

Future Directions

Despite the challenges and limitations, personalized medicine has the potential to revolutionize mental health care by providing targeted, effective, and individualized treatment options. As research and technology continue to advance, there are several exciting avenues for future exploration in the field of personalized medicine in mental health:

- **Development of biomarkers:** Researchers are actively working to identify and validate biomarkers that can serve as indicators of mental health disorders or treatment response. These biomarkers may include genetic markers, neuroimaging findings, or biochemical measurements. By incorporating biomarkers into personalized medicine approaches, clinicians can make more accurate predictions about treatment outcomes and fine-tune interventions accordingly.

- **Integration of artificial intelligence (AI):** AI and machine learning algorithms hold great potential for analyzing vast amounts of data and identifying patterns that may not be immediately evident to human clinicians. By harnessing AI technology, personalized medicine approaches can become more sophisticated and effective, helping clinicians make data-driven treatment decisions based on an individual's unique characteristics and profile.

- **Collaboration and interdisciplinary research:** Personalized medicine in mental health requires collaboration between researchers, clinicians, geneticists, neuroscientists, and other healthcare professionals. By fostering interdisciplinary collaborations, researchers can pool their expertise, share resources, and accelerate advances in personalized medicine approaches. This collaboration can also help bridge gaps between research and clinical practice, ensuring that personalized medicine tools and interventions are effectively translated into routine care settings.

- **Ethical considerations:** As personalized medicine becomes more prominent in mental health care, it is crucial to address ethical considerations surrounding privacy, informed consent, and genetic discrimination. Comprehensive guidelines and ethical frameworks should be developed to ensure that the implementation of personalized medicine approaches in mental health is guided by principles of fairness, autonomy, and respect for individual rights.

Conclusion

Personalized medicine represents a paradigm shift in mental health care, moving away from a one-size-fits-all approach towards tailored interventions that consider an individual's unique characteristics and needs. By integrating genetic information and other relevant factors, personalized medicine has the potential to improve treatment outcomes, minimize adverse drug reactions, and optimize the overall well-being of individuals with mental health disorders.

While the field of personalized medicine in mental health is still evolving, its principles and practices hold great promise for the future of mental health care. By embracing ongoing research, technological advancements, and interdisciplinary collaboration, mental health professionals can work towards a transformed landscape where personalized medicine becomes an integral part of routine clinical practice. Through this approach, we can strive to provide the highest quality of care, tailored to each individual's journey towards mental well-being.

Technology-Driven Innovation in Mental Health Care

Technology is rapidly transforming various aspects of our lives, and the field of mental health care is no exception. In recent years, there has been a surge in the development and utilization of technology-driven innovations to enhance mental health care delivery, improve access to services, and empower individuals in their own mental well-being journey. This section explores some of the key technologies that are revolutionizing the way mental health care is practiced and experienced.

Telehealth and Telemedicine

Telehealth and telemedicine have become increasingly popular in the mental health field, especially in the context of remote or underserved areas. These technologies leverage communication tools such as video conferencing, phone calls, or text-based platforms to connect individuals with mental health professionals from anywhere at any time.

One of the main advantages of telehealth is its ability to break down geographical barriers and increase access to mental health services. It eliminates the need for individuals to travel long distances for appointments, especially for those living in rural areas with limited mental health resources. Telehealth also allows individuals to receive care from the comfort and privacy of their own homes, reducing transportation and childcare-related challenges.

Moreover, telehealth can help overcome some of the stigma associated with seeking mental health care. By providing a more discreet and convenient means of accessing services, individuals may feel more comfortable reaching out for help. Additionally, virtual appointments may be less intimidating for individuals with social anxiety or agoraphobia who may find it difficult to attend in-person sessions.

It is important to note that while telehealth offers numerous benefits, it also poses certain challenges. For instance, reliable internet connectivity and access to technology are essential for effective telehealth delivery, which may be a barrier for individuals in low-resource areas or those with limited technological proficiency.

Privacy and security concerns also need to be addressed to ensure the confidentiality of personal health information.

Virtual Reality and Augmented Reality

Virtual reality (VR) and augmented reality (AR) technologies have gained significant attention in mental health care for their potential to create immersive and interactive therapeutic experiences. VR involves using computer-generated simulations to place individuals in realistic 3D environments, while AR overlays digital content onto the real-world environment.

In the field of mental health, VR and AR are used in various contexts, such as exposure therapy for anxiety disorders, phobias, and post-traumatic stress disorder (PTSD). For example, individuals with a fear of flying can undergo VR-based exposure therapy that simulates flying scenarios, allowing them to gradually confront and overcome their fears in a controlled and safe environment. Similarly, AR can be utilized to provide real-time visual cues or instructions during certain therapy sessions, enhancing the effectiveness of the interventions.

These technologies have shown promising results in terms of improving treatment outcomes, engagement, and motivation. They can create more personalized and tailored interventions by adapting the virtual environment based on an individual's specific needs. Additionally, VR and AR provide mental health professionals with opportunities for remote supervision and training, enabling them to observe and guide therapeutic sessions in real-time.

However, the high cost of VR and AR equipment, as well as the required technical expertise to develop and implement these interventions, can be significant barriers to widespread adoption. Further research is needed to explore the long-term effectiveness of these technologies and their integration into routine mental health care.

Wearable Devices and Apps

The ubiquity of smartphones and wearable devices has opened up new possibilities for mental health monitoring and support. These devices can track various physiological and behavioral markers, allowing individuals to gain insights into their mental well-being and make informed decisions about their health.

Wearable devices, such as smartwatches or fitness bands with built-in sensors, can monitor factors like heart rate, sleep patterns, and physical activity levels. By analyzing these data points, individuals can identify patterns and correlations with their mental health symptoms or triggers. This self-tracking can empower individuals to proactively manage their mental health by incorporating lifestyle changes or seeking professional support when needed.

Mental health apps have also become popular tools for self-help and support. These apps offer a wide range of features, including mood tracking, meditation exercises, cognitive behavioral therapy techniques, and educational resources. They provide individuals with accessible and convenient resources for managing their mental well-being, anytime and anywhere.

While wearable devices and mental health apps offer numerous benefits, there are important considerations to keep in mind. The accuracy and reliability of the data collected by these devices and apps may vary, and they should not replace a comprehensive clinical assessment by a qualified mental health professional. Privacy and data security are also crucial aspects to address, as individuals may be sharing sensitive information through these technologies.

Integrating Technology with Traditional Approaches

The integration of technology-driven innovations with traditional mental health care approaches holds immense potential for enhancing the effectiveness and efficiency of interventions. For instance, cognitive behavioral therapy (CBT), a widely used therapeutic approach, can be augmented with mobile apps to deliver exercises, provide reminders, and track progress. This allows individuals to engage in therapy beyond the confines of therapy sessions, reinforcing the skills and strategies they learn during treatment.

Similarly, sensor-based technologies can provide real-time feedback during exposure therapy sessions, enabling individuals and therapists to monitor and adjust the intensity of the exposure stimulus. This enhances the precision and effectiveness of the therapy, promoting better treatment outcomes.

Furthermore, technology-driven innovations can facilitate remote monitoring, enabling mental health professionals to assess treatment progress, identify potential relapses or crises, and intervene timely. By leveraging digital platforms, therapists can offer ongoing support and guidance to individuals outside of regular appointments, thereby augmenting the continuity of care.

In conclusion, technology-driven innovations are transforming mental health care by increasing access to services, enhancing treatment outcomes, and empowering individuals in their mental well-being journey. Telehealth, virtual reality, augmented reality, wearable devices, and mental health apps represent just a few examples of the many technological advancements shaping the future of mental health care. It is essential for mental health professionals to stay informed about these innovations, understand their potential benefits, and critically evaluate their use in practice. Embracing technology can unlock new opportunities for improving mental health care delivery, while ensuring that human connection and compassionate care remain at the forefront of the mental health field.

Exercises

1. Reflect on your own experiences with technology-driven mental health interventions. Have you ever used a mental health app or wearable device? How did it impact your well-being? Share your insights and discuss any challenges or limitations you encountered.

2. Imagine you are a mental health professional working in a remote area with limited access to mental health services. How could you leverage telehealth and virtual reality technologies to enhance the care you provide to individuals in your community? Discuss the potential benefits and challenges of implementing these technologies in your practice.

3. Conduct a literature review on the use of augmented reality in the treatment of specific mental health conditions, such as social anxiety disorder or obsessive-compulsive disorder. Summarize the key findings and discuss the potential applications of augmented reality in these contexts.

4. Explore different mental health apps available for smartphones. Evaluate their features, user reviews, and evidence base. Select one app that you believe could be beneficial for a specific population or mental health condition. Develop a brief proposal outlining how this app could be integrated into a mental health treatment program.

5. Research the ethical considerations surrounding the use of wearable devices and mental health apps. Identify potential privacy and data security risks and discuss strategies for mitigating them. Consider the implications for informed consent and patient autonomy.

Resources

- American Telemedicine Association: www.americantelemed.org - Virtual Reality Medical Center: www.vrphobia.com - National Institute of Mental Health: www.nimh.nih.gov - PsyberGuide: www.psyberguide.org - Digital Mental Health: www.digitalmentalhealth.uk

The Role of Peer Support in Mental Health

Peer support plays a crucial role in promoting mental health and well-being. It refers to the provision of emotional, social, and informational support from individuals who have shared experiences or similar backgrounds. Peer support can take many forms, such as peer counseling, peer mentoring, and peer-led support groups. In this section, we will explore the significance of peer support in mental health, its benefits, and how it can be integrated into mental health care.

Understanding Peer Support

Peer support is grounded in the belief that individuals who have gone through similar experiences can offer unique insights and guidance to others facing similar challenges. It is based on the principles of empathy, shared understanding, and mutual respect. Peer support provides a non-judgmental space where individuals can openly share their thoughts and feelings without fear of stigma or discrimination.

Peer support can be particularly beneficial for individuals with mental health concerns. It recognizes that mental health issues can be isolating and that connecting with peers who have faced similar struggles can foster a sense of belonging and validation. Additionally, peer support offers an alternative or complement to traditional mental health services by providing informal, accessible, and community-based support.

Benefits of Peer Support

1. Empowerment and Self-Determination: Peer support empowers individuals by promoting self-determination and autonomy over their own recovery journey. Peers can provide hope, encouragement, and practical strategies that promote personal growth and well-being.

2. Shared Lived Experience: Peers who have successfully navigated their own mental health challenges can offer invaluable insight, empathy, and understanding. Sharing experiences helps individuals realize that they are not alone and that recovery is possible.

3. Building Social Connections: Peer support facilitates the development of social connections and a sense of community. It reduces feelings of isolation and loneliness, which are common among individuals with mental health concerns.

4. Reduced Stigma: Peers who openly discuss their experiences challenge stereotypes and reduce stigma surrounding mental health. By sharing personal stories, they contribute to a more inclusive and understanding society, promoting acceptance and compassion.

5. Increased Treatment Engagement: Peer support can enhance treatment engagement and adherence. Peers can offer practical guidance on navigating mental

health services, provide emotional support during challenging times, and help individuals stay motivated on their recovery journey.

Integrating Peer Support into Mental Health Care

To fully realize the potential of peer support in mental health care, it is essential to integrate it into existing service models. Here are some strategies for incorporating peer support:

1. Peer Support Specialists: Mental health service organizations can hire trained peer support specialists who have lived experience with mental health challenges. These specialists can work alongside other mental health professionals, providing guidance, advocacy, and support to individuals receiving care.

2. Peer-Led Support Groups: Establishing peer-led support groups provides a safe and supportive environment for individuals to share experiences and learn from one another. These groups can be focused on specific mental health concerns (e.g., depression, anxiety) or cater to specific populations (e.g., veterans, LGBTQ+ individuals).

3. Peer Mentoring Programs: Peer mentoring programs pair individuals with peers who have successfully managed their mental health challenges. Mentors offer guidance, encouragement, and support as mentees work towards their recovery goals.

4. Peer-Run Organizations: Supporting and funding peer-run organizations that provide a range of peer support services is crucial. These organizations can offer peer-led programs, advocacy, education, and resources to the wider community.

It is important to note that while peer support can be highly effective, it is not a substitute for professional mental health treatment. Peer support should complement and be integrated into a comprehensive mental health care plan.

Real-World Example: Peer Support in the Recovery Journey

Let's consider a real-world example to illustrate the role of peer support in mental health. Sarah, a young woman experiencing symptoms of bipolar disorder, joins a peer-led support group focused on mood disorders. In this group, she meets peers who understand her experiences and can offer practical strategies for symptom management.

Sarah forms connections with others in the group and feels a sense of validation and acceptance. Through peer support, she gains hope and begins to see that recovery is possible. Sarah also learns about local resources and treatment options from her peers, which helps her navigate the complex mental health system with more confidence.

Over time, Sarah becomes an active member of the group, sharing her own experiences and offering support to others who are in earlier stages of their recovery journey. Through peer support, Sarah not only receives the help she needs but also becomes an agent of change, promoting mental health and well-being in her community.

Conclusion

Peer support has a vital role to play in the mental health landscape. By harnessing the power of shared experiences and fostering a sense of community, peer support can empower individuals, reduce stigma, and enhance the overall well-being of those with mental health concerns. Integrating peer support into mental health care models and providing resources for peer-led initiatives are essential steps in building a more comprehensive, inclusive, and effective approach to mental health and well-being.

A Call for Action: Advocacy and Policy in Mental Health

The Importance of Advocacy to Effect Change

Advocacy plays a crucial role in the field of mental health, as it is a powerful tool for effecting change at both the individual and societal level. By advocating for improved access to mental health services, better policies, and reduced stigma, advocates contribute to creating a society that supports the mental well-being of all its members. In this section, we will explore the importance of advocacy in promoting positive change in mental health, and we will discuss strategies for effective advocacy.

The Need for Advocacy in Mental Health

Mental health issues affect a significant portion of the global population, yet access to quality mental health care remains limited in many parts of the world. Stigma and discrimination further compound the challenges faced by individuals seeking help for their mental well-being. In such a landscape, advocacy becomes essential to ensure that the rights and needs of individuals with mental health difficulties are addressed.

Advocacy is crucial in challenging the pervasive stigma associated with mental illness. Advocates work to change societal perceptions and attitudes towards mental health through education and awareness campaigns. By promoting understanding and empathy, advocacy efforts can help reduce the discrimination often faced by individuals with mental health challenges.

Moreover, advocacy is essential for influencing public policy and resource allocation. By raising awareness about the gaps in mental health care and the impact of policies on individuals with mental health difficulties, advocates can advocate for improved access to services, increased funding, and the development of evidence-based policies. In this way, advocacy aims to create a more supportive and inclusive mental health care system.

Strategies for Effective Advocacy

To effectively advocate for change in the field of mental health, advocates must employ various strategies and approaches. Here are some key strategies for effective advocacy:

1. Building coalitions and partnerships: Collaboration with like-minded organizations and individuals amplifies the impact of advocacy efforts. By joining forces, advocates can pool resources, knowledge, and expertise to create a stronger voice for change.

2. Strategic communication and messaging: Advocacy efforts must be accompanied by effective communication strategies. Developing clear and compelling messages, backed by evidence and personal stories, can help raise awareness and change public opinion.

3. Engaging policymakers and stakeholders: Advocates must actively engage with policymakers, healthcare providers, and other relevant stakeholders to ensure that their concerns and perspectives are heard. This involves participating in policy discussions, attending public hearings, and building relationships with key decision-makers.

4. Empowering individuals with lived experience: People with personal experience of mental health difficulties can be powerful advocates. Empowering individuals to share their stories, providing them with the necessary skills and platforms, and ensuring their voices are heard are essential elements of effective advocacy.

5. Grassroots initiatives and mobilization: Local and community-based advocacy efforts can make a significant impact. By organizing grassroots initiatives such as awareness campaigns, support groups, and community events, advocates

can engage directly with individuals and communities, fostering a sense of solidarity and driving local change.

6. Monitoring and evaluation: Advocacy efforts should be regularly assessed and evaluated to measure their impact and effectiveness. Monitoring the progress of advocacy initiatives allows advocates to adapt their strategies, identify areas for improvement, and ensure that their efforts contribute to meaningful change.

Real-World Example: The Mental Health Parity and Addiction Equity Act

An excellent example of effective advocacy leading to significant change is the Mental Health Parity and Addiction Equity Act (MHPAEA) in the United States. This legislation, passed in 2008, requires health insurance plans to provide equal coverage for mental health and substance use disorders as they do for physical health conditions. The law ensures that insurance companies cannot impose stricter limits on mental health benefits or charge higher co-pays compared to medical and surgical benefits.

The MHPAEA was the result of years of advocacy by mental health organizations, advocates, and individuals with lived experience. Through grassroots initiatives, lobbying efforts, and the sharing of personal stories, advocates successfully conveyed the importance of equitable mental health coverage to lawmakers. As a result, millions of Americans gained improved access to mental health care, reducing financial barriers and increasing the overall quality of mental health services.

Ethical Considerations and Challenges

Advocacy in mental health also faces ethical considerations and challenges. Advocates must ensure that their efforts respect the autonomy and privacy of individuals with mental health difficulties. Sharing personal stories should be done with the individual's informed consent, and efforts must be made to protect their confidentiality and well-being.

Additionally, advocacy efforts should be based on accurate information and supported by evidence-based research. By grounding their arguments in solid evidence, advocates can ensure that their message is credible and persuasive.

It is also essential for advocates to acknowledge and address the power dynamics inherent in advocacy work. They must strive to include diverse voices and perspectives, particularly those of marginalized communities, to ensure that advocacy efforts are inclusive and representative.

Conclusion

Advocacy is a vital tool in promoting positive change in the field of mental health. By advocating for improved access to services, reduced stigma, and effective policies, advocates contribute to creating a more equitable and supportive society for individuals with mental health difficulties. Through strategic approaches, effective communication, and collaborations, advocates can effect meaningful change in mental health care systems and improve the well-being of individuals worldwide.

Empowering individuals, engaging policymakers, and fostering grassroots initiatives are key strategies for effective advocacy. By employing these approaches and addressing ethical considerations, advocates can drive change, challenge the status quo, and create a future that prioritizes mental health and well-being.

Exercises

1. Reflect on a personal experience or observation related to mental health stigma. Discuss how you can use advocacy to challenge and change those attitudes.

2. Explore local mental health organizations or initiatives in your community. Identify ways in which you can contribute to or support their advocacy efforts.

3. Research a current mental health policy or legislation in your country. Evaluate its impact on accessibility and equity in mental health care. Consider potential areas for improvement and possible advocacy efforts to address these issues.

4. Develop a persuasive message or campaign to raise awareness about the importance of mental health parity in insurance coverage. Consider the key arguments, evidence, and messaging strategies that would resonate with various audiences.

5. Form a small advocacy group with your peers to address a specific mental health issue in your community or school. Develop a plan of action, including strategies for engagement, communication, and evaluation of your advocacy efforts.

Policy Considerations for Promoting Mental Health and Wellbeing

Developing effective policies is crucial in promoting mental health and wellbeing at both individual and societal levels. This section explores key policy considerations that can contribute to positive mental health outcomes. These considerations aim to address the complex nature of mental health and foster a supportive environment for individuals to thrive.

1. Integration of Mental Health in Public Health Policies

One of the fundamental policy considerations is the integration of mental health into broader public health policies. Mental health should be recognized as an integral component of overall well-being and should receive equal attention as physical health. Policies should emphasize the importance of prevention, early intervention, and the reduction of risk factors associated with mental health problems.

For example, policies can focus on promoting mental health literacy by incorporating mental health education in schools, workplaces, and community settings. By increasing awareness and knowledge about mental health, individuals can be empowered to recognize the early signs of mental health issues and seek appropriate support.

2. Access to Mental Health Services

Policy initiatives should prioritize equitable access to mental health services for all individuals. Disparities in accessing mental health care exist due to various factors such as income, geographic location, ethnicity, and social stigma. Policies should aim to reduce these barriers and ensure that mental health services are accessible, affordable, and culturally sensitive.

To achieve this, policies can include measures such as expanding the mental health workforce, increasing funding for mental health services, and implementing telehealth initiatives. Telehealth can bridge the gap between individuals in remote areas and mental health professionals, allowing for timely and convenient access to care.

3. Collaboration Across Sectors

Addressing mental health challenges requires a collaborative approach across various sectors, including healthcare, education, employment, and social welfare. Policies should encourage intersectoral collaboration to ensure a holistic and integrated response to mental health issues.

For instance, policies can promote partnerships between healthcare providers and schools to implement mental health programs for students. By integrating mental health into the education system, early identification of mental health issues can occur, leading to timely interventions and support.

4. Addressing Social Determinants of Mental Health

Social determinants of mental health, such as poverty, discrimination, and social exclusion, significantly impact mental health outcomes. Policies should address these determinants to create an environment that promotes mental health and reduces the risk of mental illness.

Policy initiatives can focus on poverty reduction measures, promoting social inclusion, and combating discrimination. Additionally, policies can support the provision of safe and affordable housing, employment opportunities, and supportive social networks, all of which contribute to positive mental health outcomes.

5. Prevention and Early Intervention

Prevention and early intervention are key pillars of effective mental health policies. Policies should prioritize prevention strategies that target the promotion of mental well-being and the prevention of mental health problems before they escalate.

Promoting mental health literacy, implementing anti-stigma campaigns, and providing early intervention services are effective strategies. Policies can support the integration of mental health screening and early intervention services in primary care settings, ensuring that individuals receive timely support.

6. Data-Informed Decision Making

Policy decisions should be guided by accurate data, research, and evidence. Policies should support the collection and analysis of data on mental health prevalence, service utilization, and outcomes to inform decision making and resource allocation.

Furthermore, policies can prioritize research funding to advance our understanding of mental health and develop evidence-based interventions. By ensuring that policies are based on reliable evidence, we can improve the effectiveness and efficiency of mental health promotion efforts.

7. Advocacy and Awareness

Policy considerations should include provisions for advocacy and awareness campaigns to reduce stigma and promote mental health. Policies can encourage the active involvement of mental health service users, families, and community organizations in policy development and implementation.

By amplifying the voices of those with lived experience and involving them in decision making, policies can better reflect the needs of the population. Additionally, policies can allocate resources to support community-driven mental health initiatives and empower individuals and communities to take an active role in promoting mental health.

In conclusion, policy considerations play a vital role in promoting mental health and wellbeing. By integrating mental health into public health policies, ensuring access to services, promoting collaboration, addressing social determinants, emphasizing prevention and early intervention, using data-informed decision making, and supporting advocacy and awareness, policies can create an environment conducive to positive mental health outcomes. It is through thoughtful and comprehensive policies that we can shape a transformed mental health landscape for the future.

Strategies for Empowering Individuals and Communities

Empowering individuals and communities is a crucial step in promoting mental health and wellbeing. It involves providing people with the knowledge, tools, and support they need to take control of their own mental health and make positive changes in their lives. In this section, we will discuss some effective strategies for empowering individuals and communities in the context of mental health.

1. Education and Awareness

Education and awareness play a vital role in empowering individuals and communities. By increasing knowledge and understanding of mental health and wellbeing, people can make informed decisions about their own mental health and seek appropriate support when needed.

One strategy is to provide community workshops and training programs that aim to educate individuals about mental health issues, common mental disorders, and available resources. These workshops can be conducted by mental health professionals, community leaders, or even individuals with lived experience of mental health challenges. By disseminating accurate information and debunking myths and misconceptions, these educational initiatives help reduce stigma and promote a more supportive and inclusive community.

Another important aspect of education and awareness is promoting mental health literacy. This involves improving people's understanding of mental health, including the ability to recognize the signs and symptoms of common mental disorders and respond appropriately. Mental health literacy programs can be integrated into schools, workplaces, and community organizations to ensure that individuals have the necessary skills to support themselves and those around them.

2. Peer Support Networks

Peer support networks are another valuable strategy for empowering individuals and communities. Peer support involves connecting individuals who have experienced similar mental health challenges to provide mutual support, understanding, and guidance.

Peer support networks can take various forms, including support groups, online communities, and mentorship programs. These networks foster a sense of belonging, reduce isolation, and provide individuals with a safe space to share their experiences and learn from others. Through peer support, individuals gain a sense of hope, resilience, and empowerment as they witness others overcoming their own mental health challenges.

It is important to ensure that peer support networks are accessible and inclusive, catering to diverse populations and specific mental health needs. Educating and training peer supporters, as well as establishing clear guidelines and boundaries, is crucial for maintaining the quality and effectiveness of these networks.

3. Community Engagement and Collaboration

Empowering individuals and communities also involves fostering community engagement and collaboration. This strategy encourages active participation and involvement in mental health initiatives, promoting a sense of ownership and responsibility among community members.

One way to encourage community engagement is through the establishment of community-based organizations and initiatives. These organizations can work collaboratively with mental health professionals, educators, policymakers, and other stakeholders to develop and implement strategies that address the unique needs of the community.

Additionally, involving individuals with lived experience of mental health challenges in the planning and decision-making processes is essential. Their perspectives and insights can inform the development of more effective and inclusive mental health interventions.

Collaboration with different sectors, such as healthcare, education, employment, and housing, is also crucial in empowering individuals and communities. By working together, these sectors can create supportive environments and address the social determinants of mental health. For example, collaboration between mental health services and schools can promote early intervention and provide appropriate support to students experiencing mental health difficulties.

4. Advocacy and Policy Change

Advocacy and policy change are powerful strategies for empowering individuals and communities in the realm of mental health. Through advocacy, individuals and organizations can work to change policies and practices that hinder mental health promotion and access to quality services.

Advocacy can take many forms, including raising awareness about specific mental health issues, challenging stigma and discrimination, and promoting the rights of individuals with mental health challenges. It involves engaging with policymakers, media outlets, and the general public to create change at the societal level.

Policy change is a critical aspect of advocacy, as it has the potential to transform mental health systems and resources. This can involve advocating for increased funding for mental health services, improving access to care, and promoting policies that prioritize prevention and early intervention. By working towards policy change, individuals and communities can create a more supportive and inclusive mental health landscape.

5. Building Resilience and Coping Skills

Empowering individuals and communities also involves helping them build resilience and develop effective coping skills. Resilience is the ability to bounce back from adversity, and it plays a crucial role in promoting mental health and wellbeing.

One strategy for building resilience is providing individuals with tools and techniques to manage stress and improve their emotional wellbeing. This can include mindfulness exercises, relaxation techniques, and stress management training. By equipping individuals with these skills, they become better equipped to navigate challenges and maintain good mental health.

Additionally, promoting positive coping mechanisms, such as regular physical activity, healthy eating, and creative outlets, can empower individuals to take proactive steps towards their mental wellbeing. These activities not only provide a sense of purpose and fulfillment but also serve as protective factors against the development of mental health disorders.

Conclusion

Empowering individuals and communities is a fundamental aspect of promoting mental health and wellbeing. By implementing strategies such as education and awareness, peer support networks, community engagement and collaboration, advocacy and policy change, and building resilience and coping skills, we can create a more inclusive and supportive mental health landscape.

It is important to remember that empowering individuals and communities is an ongoing process that requires ongoing commitment and collaboration. By working together, we can create a future where mental health is prioritized, stigma is eliminated, and everyone has access to the support they need to lead fulfilling lives. Let us be the agents of change and transform mental health care for the better.

Conclusion: Shaping a Transformed Mental Health Landscape

Reflection on the Transformative Approaches Explored

As we conclude our exploration of transformative approaches to mental health and wellbeing, it is essential to reflect on the impact and significance of these innovative techniques, holistic strategies, and cutting-edge research. Through this journey, we have gained a deeper understanding of the complex nature of mental health and the various methods that can shape the future of wellness.

The transformative approaches we have examined offer a departure from traditional biomedical models and emphasize a holistic and integrative perspective. They recognize the interconnectedness of the mind, body, and spirit and underscore the importance of addressing the unique needs and experiences of individuals in their cultural and contextual contexts.

One major theme that emerged from our exploration is the power of therapeutic techniques such as Cognitive Behavioral Therapy (CBT), mindfulness-based interventions, art therapy, and expressive writing. These approaches provide individuals with tools and strategies to navigate their thoughts, emotions, and behaviors. By actively engaging with these techniques, individuals can gain insight, develop coping mechanisms, and find empowerment in their journey towards improved mental health and wellbeing.

For instance, CBT has proven to be effective in treating various mental health disorders, such as anxiety, depression, and addiction. By challenging negative and distorted thoughts, individuals can reframe their thinking patterns and cultivate healthier beliefs and behaviors.

Mindfulness-based interventions have also gained considerable attention for their ability to cultivate present-moment awareness, reduce stress, and enhance overall wellbeing. The practice of mindfulness encourages individuals to observe their thoughts and emotions without judgment, promoting a deeper understanding of one's inner experiences and fostering self-compassion.

Art therapy offers a unique and expressive approach to mental health by harnessing the creative process. Through various artistic mediums, individuals can access and express emotions that may be difficult to verbalize. This form of therapy allows for the exploration of personal narratives, and the creation of visual representations can be a powerful catalyst for healing and self-discovery.

Similarly, expressive writing can serve as a therapeutic tool for individuals to explore their thoughts, emotions, and experiences in a structured and reflective manner. By putting pen to paper, individuals can gain clarity, process trauma, and find relief from emotional distress.

In addition to these individual therapeutic techniques, we have also explored the importance of holistic strategies for mental health and wellbeing. Nutrition, exercise, sleep, social support, and self-care practices have proven instrumental in creating a strong foundation for mental wellness.

For example, the gut-brain connection reminds us of the significant impact that nutrition can have on mental health. Consuming a balanced diet rich in nutrients supports brain function and can positively influence mood and cognitive performance.

Regular exercise and physical activity have been associated with reduced symptoms of depression and anxiety. Engaging in different types of exercise not only improves physical fitness but also enhances mood, boosts self-esteem, and provides a sense of accomplishment.

Sleep, often overlooked, is a vital component of mental wellbeing. Quality sleep is essential for cognitive functioning, emotional regulation, and overall mental health. By adopting healthy sleep habits and practicing good sleep hygiene, individuals can optimize their mental wellness.

Equally important is the role of social support and connection in mental health. Cultivating strong and supportive relationships, both within personal networks and the broader community, is crucial for emotional wellbeing. Building a sense of belonging and engaging in meaningful social interactions provide a buffer against stress and contribute to overall happiness and life satisfaction.

Lastly, self-care practices empower individuals to prioritize their own wellbeing. Self-care is the intentional practice of activities that promote physical, emotional, and mental health. By incorporating self-care into daily routines and establishing personalized self-care practices, individuals can nourish their mind, body, and spirit.

Our exploration of transformative approaches would be incomplete without acknowledging the exciting advancements in research and technology that are shaping the future of mental health and wellbeing. Neuroscience, as a rapidly evolving field, has offered valuable insights into the intricate workings of the brain and its connection to mental health. Techniques such as neuroimaging have allowed researchers to visualize brain activity and gain a better understanding of the neural mechanisms underlying mental health disorders.

Innovative technologies, such as telehealth, virtual reality, augmented reality, and wearable devices, have opened up new avenues for mental health care and support. These technologies provide opportunities for remote access to mental health services, immersive therapeutic experiences, and personalized monitoring of mental health indicators. They have the potential to increase the reach and effectiveness of mental health care, allowing for greater accessibility and tailoring of interventions to individual needs.

Another emerging area of research that holds promise for mental health treatment is psychedelics-assisted therapy. Recent studies have shown that substances such as psilocybin and MDMA, when used in a controlled therapeutic setting, can provide profound therapeutic effects for individuals with treatment-resistant depression, PTSD, and other mental health conditions. However, integrating these substances into mainstream mental health care requires careful consideration of ethical, legal, and safety concerns.

Epigenetics, the study of gene-environment interactions, offers an exciting perspective on the interplay between genetics and mental health. It highlights the potential impact of environmental factors on gene expression and presents opportunities for personalized treatment approaches that consider an individual's unique genetic makeup and life experiences.

Cultural considerations have also played a significant role throughout our exploration. Recognizing the influence of culture on mental health and adopting culturally sensitive approaches in research and practice are essential for providing equitable and effective care. Embracing intersectionality, which acknowledges the interconnected nature of various social identities, enables us to better understand the complex and diverse experiences of individuals and communities.

As we conclude our journey through the transformative approaches to mental health and wellbeing, it is crucial to recognize the challenges and opportunities that lie ahead. The realization of a transformed mental health landscape requires addressing systemic issues such as access and equity in mental health services, socioeconomic and structural influences on mental health, and the integration of mental health into primary care settings.

Looking forward, the future of mental health research and practice is marked by several emerging trends. Personalized medicine holds the promise of tailoring treatment approaches to individual needs based on genetic, biological, and environmental factors. Technology-driven innovation, including digital tools and artificial intelligence, will continue to shape how mental health care is delivered, monitored, and supported. Peer support will play an increasingly vital role in fostering connections, reducing isolation, and providing empathetic understanding within communities.

Advocacy and policy are instrumental in effecting change in the mental health landscape. By raising awareness, challenging stigmas, and promoting policies that prioritize mental health and wellbeing, we can create supportive environments that foster the flourishing of individuals and communities.

In conclusion, the transformative approaches explored in this book have shed light on the potential for enhancing mental health and wellbeing through innovative techniques, holistic strategies, and cutting-edge research. By adopting these approaches, we can pave the way for a future where mental health is understood, valued, and prioritized. Let us continue to inspire and be inspired by the possibilities that lie ahead, encouraging further research, innovation, and collaboration in the field of mental health.

The Potential Impact of Transformative Mental Health Care

Transformative mental health care has the potential to revolutionize the field and profoundly impact individuals, communities, and society as a whole. By embracing innovative techniques, holistic strategies, and cutting-edge research, transformative mental health care can address the current challenges and gaps in traditional approaches, leading to improved outcomes and enhanced overall well-being.

One of the key potential impacts of transformative mental health care is the shift from solely focusing on symptom management to a more comprehensive approach that emphasizes prevention and early intervention. This proactive approach can help identify mental health issues at their early stages, allowing for timely and targeted interventions that may prevent the development or worsening of mental health disorders. By addressing mental health concerns early on, transformative care can lead to better long-term outcomes and reduced healthcare costs.

Another potential impact of transformative mental health care is the reduction of stigma and discrimination surrounding mental health. Traditional approaches to mental health have often perpetuated stigmatizing attitudes and practices, contributing to the reluctance of individuals to seek help and hindering their recovery. Transformative care recognizes the importance of creating safe and inclusive environments that foster acceptance and understanding. By promoting social inclusion and challenging stigma, transformative care can encourage individuals to seek support and access necessary services without fear of judgment or discrimination.

Additionally, transformative mental health care has the potential to improve access to services and reduce disparities in mental health care. Traditional models of care have often been inaccessible or inequitable, with limited resources and services available to marginalized populations. Transformative care emphasizes the importance of equitable access to quality mental health services and strives to address the socioeconomic and structural influences that contribute to disparities. By adopting innovative technologies, such as telehealth and mobile applications, transformative care can extend mental health services beyond traditional settings, making them more accessible to underserved populations.

Furthermore, transformative mental health care can improve collaboration and integration among different disciplines within the healthcare system. Traditional approaches to mental health have often been fragmented and siloed, resulting in disjointed care and limited holistic understanding of individuals' needs. Transformative care recognizes the complex interplay between various factors that influence mental health and encourages interdisciplinary collaboration. By integrating mental health into primary care settings and promoting interdisciplinary teamwork, transformative care can provide comprehensive care that addresses the physical, psychological, and social aspects of individuals' well-being.

Lastly, transformative mental health care has the potential to empower individuals and communities. By emphasizing self-care practices, promoting peer support networks, and involving individuals in decisions regarding their care, transformative care strengthens their sense of agency and resilience. This empowerment can lead to increased self-efficacy, improved coping skills, and enhanced overall well-being. Transformative care also recognizes the importance of community and social networks in mental health, facilitating the development of supportive relationships and fostering a sense of belonging and connectedness.

In conclusion, transformative mental health care holds great promise in shaping a more inclusive, compassionate, and effective approach to mental health and well-being. Through its potential impacts, such as early intervention, reduced stigma, improved access, enhanced collaboration, and empowerment, transformative care can contribute to the creation of a transformed mental health landscape. As we continue to explore innovative techniques, holistic strategies, and cutting-edge research, it is essential to advocate for the integration of transformative care into mental health systems, policies, and practices to ensure the delivery of high-quality and person-centered care for all individuals.

Encouraging Continued Research, Innovation, and Collaboration

In order to shape a transformed mental health landscape, it is crucial to encourage continued research, innovation, and collaboration. This section explores the importance of these three components and provides strategies to promote and sustain them within the field of mental health.

The Importance of Research

Research plays a vital role in advancing our understanding of mental health and developing evidence-based interventions. By conducting rigorous studies, researchers can investigate the effectiveness of different therapeutic approaches, explore the mechanisms underlying mental health disorders, and identify factors that contribute to mental wellbeing. Continued research is essential for expanding our knowledge base and improving the quality of care provided to individuals with mental health concerns.

Example: For instance, research studies have demonstrated the effectiveness of mindfulness-based interventions in reducing symptoms of anxiety and depression. This knowledge has led to the integration of mindfulness practices into various treatment settings, benefitting individuals in their journey towards improved mental health.

To encourage continued research in mental health, various strategies can be implemented:

1. **Funding Support:** Governments, private organizations, and philanthropic entities should provide adequate funding to support mental health research initiatives. This includes allocating resources for large-scale longitudinal studies, clinical trials, and interdisciplinary collaborations. By prioritizing research funding, we can incentivize scientists and clinicians to pursue innovative projects and make significant contributions to the field.

2. **Research Mentoring Programs:** Establishing mentoring programs that pair experienced researchers with early career professionals can foster a culture of continuous learning and skill development. These mentorship relationships provide guidance and support, encouraging young researchers to pursue ambitious projects and navigate the complex research landscape.

3. **Dissemination of Findings:** It is crucial to disseminate research findings to the scientific community, mental health practitioners, policy-makers, and the general public. This can be achieved through publications in scientific journals, conference presentations, and accessible summaries of research findings. By communicating research outcomes effectively, we can facilitate the translation of knowledge into practice and influence policy decisions.

The Power of Innovation

Innovation brings fresh perspectives, novel ideas, and creative solutions to the field of mental health. It involves developing new models of care, exploring alternative treatment approaches, and leveraging technological advancements to enhance interventions. Embracing innovation can lead to breakthroughs in mental health research, improve the effectiveness of interventions, and increase access to care.

Example: Virtual reality (VR) technology has emerged as a promising tool in the treatment of anxiety disorders. VR-based exposure therapy allows individuals to safely confront their fears and overcome phobias in a controlled and immersive environment. This innovative approach has shown promising results and has the potential to revolutionize mental health care.

To foster a culture of innovation in mental health, the following strategies can be adopted:

1. **Collaboration with Technology Experts:** Mental health professionals should collaborate with experts in technology, such as virtual reality developers, app designers, and data scientists. Through interdisciplinary collaborations, innovative technologies and digital solutions can be developed to address mental health needs and increase treatment accessibility.

2. **Support for Start-ups and Entrepreneurship:** Creating an ecosystem that supports mental health start-ups and entrepreneurship can stimulate innovation within the field. Providing resources, mentorship, and funding opportunities specifically targeted at mental health innovation can encourage individuals to develop and implement groundbreaking ideas in mental health care.

3. **Exploring Non-traditional Approaches:** Embracing non-traditional approaches, such as alternative therapies, mind-body practices, and complementary interventions, can foster innovation in mental health. By investigating unconventional techniques and exploring their potential

benefits, we can expand the range of treatments available and cater to diverse individual needs.

The Value of Collaboration

Collaboration lies at the heart of transforming mental health care. By fostering partnerships and collaboration among researchers, practitioners, policymakers, and individuals with lived experiences, we can enhance the collective understanding of mental health and develop comprehensive, person-centered approaches to care.

Example: The Recovery-Oriented Approach, which emphasizes an individual's strengths, choices, and goals, was developed through collaboration between mental health professionals and individuals with lived experiences. This collaborative effort has resulted in a paradigm shift towards more empowering and inclusive mental health care.

To promote collaboration in mental health, consider the following strategies:

1. **Interdisciplinary and Cross-Sector Collaboration:** Encouraging collaboration among professionals from diverse disciplines, such as psychology, psychiatry, social work, nursing, and occupational therapy, can lead to holistic and comprehensive care. Additionally, collaboration with representatives from education, employment, housing, and justice sectors can address social determinants of mental health and improve overall wellbeing.

2. **Patient and Family Engagement:** Involving individuals with lived experiences, as well as their families and support networks, in the planning, implementation, and evaluation of mental health services is crucial. Their unique insights can inform the development of more person-centered and culturally responsive interventions.

3. **International Partnerships:** Collaboration on a global scale can drive innovation and exchange of best practices in mental health care. International partnerships can facilitate the sharing of culturally specific knowledge and enhance our understanding of mental health disparities and needs across diverse populations.

By promoting continued research, innovation, and collaboration, we can shape a transformed mental health landscape that is inclusive, effective, and person-centered. Through these collective efforts, we can improve mental health outcomes, reduce stigma, and ensure the well-being of individuals and communities. Let us forge ahead with determination and embrace the challenges and opportunities that lie ahead.

Index

-doubt, 48
-effectiveness, 147

ability, 1, 2, 6, 7, 34, 35, 41, 49, 55, 56, 60, 85, 100, 127–129, 149, 169, 181, 183, 185
ableism, 20
Abraham Maslow, 4
absence, 1, 11
abuse, 93, 137
acceptability, 157
acceptance, 4, 9, 10, 34, 48, 55, 93, 98–100, 105, 173, 174, 188
access, 5, 8–10, 13, 44, 48, 74, 98, 100, 107, 118, 119, 127, 128, 130, 131, 137, 147, 148, 150, 151, 157–162, 164, 167, 169, 171, 172, 175–179, 181, 183–186, 188, 190
accessibility, 19, 116, 124, 128, 129, 135, 139, 167, 178, 186
accomplishment, 83, 185
account, 14, 45, 117, 146, 165, 166
accountability, 74, 82, 83, 108
accuracy, 130, 150, 171
acetylation, 139, 140

achievement, 82
act, 1, 43, 61, 63, 73, 93, 100, 107
action, 13, 94, 95, 134, 178
activation, 87, 113
activity, 45, 54, 67, 73, 75, 76, 81, 82, 86, 101, 114, 115, 117, 143, 170, 183, 185, 186
actualization, 4, 39
adaptability, 59
addiction, 34, 115, 139, 142, 184
addition, 24, 63, 69, 71, 129, 139, 185
adherence, 20, 93, 130, 148–150, 173
adjunct, 42, 75, 135
adoption, 147, 170
advance, 114, 145, 167, 180
advancement, 138
adversity, 93, 100, 144, 183
advice, 92, 96
advocacy, 5, 9, 95, 98, 159, 161, 174–178, 180, 181, 183, 184
advocate, 10, 150, 153, 162, 176, 189
affirmation, 93
affordability, 135, 157
age, 1, 50, 73, 94

agency, 57, 63, 188
agent, 175
agoraphobia, 169
aid, 55
aim, 17–19, 39, 178, 179, 181
air, 80, 144
alcohol, 34
alertness, 85
alignment, 51
alliance, 150
allocation, 164, 176, 180
alternative, 16, 24, 25, 47, 63, 133, 137, 167, 173, 190
amber, 90
amygdala, 112
analysis, 116, 154, 180
anger, 58
animal, 18, 19
anthropology, 2
antioxidant, 68
anxiety, 6, 7, 17, 25, 26, 33, 43, 47, 48, 54, 55, 58, 61, 63, 65, 66, 68, 70, 73, 74, 76, 79, 84, 85, 87–90, 92–94, 96, 99, 113, 118, 126, 127, 133, 136, 139, 142, 143, 169, 172, 184, 185
apnea, 87, 89
app, 172
appetite, 25
application, 28, 29, 129
appointment, 81
appraisal, 93, 95
appreciation, 97, 98
approach, 2, 3, 5, 7, 9, 12–18, 21, 24, 27, 28, 41, 44–46, 48–51, 55, 56, 59, 62, 67–70, 79, 80, 94, 95, 117, 118, 131, 133, 135, 136, 142, 145–147, 149, 153, 158, 161–166, 168, 169, 175, 179, 185, 187, 188
appropriateness, 157
appropriation, 56
area, 90, 118, 172, 186
arousal, 59
array, 65
art, 14, 39, 41–48
artery, 6
artwork, 45, 48
aspect, 2, 15, 17, 18, 28, 54, 80, 85–87, 96, 101, 104–107, 135, 181, 183, 184
assertiveness, 99
assessment, 23, 69, 120, 150, 163, 171
assistance, 92, 93, 96, 98, 159
association, 83
attention, 8, 13, 29, 33, 35, 42, 55, 69, 73, 80, 84, 90, 97, 106, 120, 124, 132, 142, 179, 185
attitude, 29, 69
attribution, 20
autism, 65, 118, 127
autonomy, 114, 155, 172, 173, 177
availability, 19, 116, 157, 159, 161, 167
awareness, 2, 4, 9, 10, 17, 20, 21, 29, 33–36, 42, 43, 48–51, 55, 57, 58, 60, 80, 98, 128, 134, 149, 150, 159, 176, 178–181, 183–185, 187
axis, 65, 66, 118, 119
axon, 112

background, 1, 17, 157
backlash, 132

bacteria, 66, 67
balance, 3, 21, 49, 54, 80, 84, 100, 101, 114
barrier, 11, 66, 107, 108, 116, 163, 169
base, 135, 172, 189
basic, 8
basis, 117, 146
bath, 86, 90
bed, 85, 86, 89, 90
bedroom, 85, 90
bedtime, 86, 88–90
beef, 68
beginner, 51
beginning, 51
behavior, 4, 23, 65
behavioral, 14, 17, 23, 24, 26, 28, 39, 59, 129, 170, 171
being, 1–7, 9, 11, 15, 16, 27–32, 34, 38, 39, 41, 43, 48–56, 58, 62, 63, 67, 69, 70, 80, 82, 83, 85–89, 92, 97–99, 101, 103, 104, 106–108, 114, 127–131, 133, 135–137, 139, 140, 142–145, 148, 150, 151, 153–155, 165, 168–173, 175, 177–180, 187, 188, 191
belief, 27, 107, 173
belonging, 6, 7, 15, 82, 92–94, 97–100, 173, 182, 185, 188
benefit, 17, 24, 69, 135, 146
bike, 74
biking, 81, 82
Bikram, 50
Bikram Yoga, 50
binge, 26
biofeedback, 128

biology, 3, 113, 141–143
blackout, 90
blood, 6, 55, 58, 66, 73, 82, 146, 167
bloodstream, 115
body, 15–17, 26, 33, 34, 36, 49, 51–56, 68, 73, 74, 76, 78–80, 85, 89, 90, 112, 129, 184, 186
bodyweight, 74, 77
bond, 97
book, 75, 86, 90, 95, 187
boost, 74
brain, 4, 11, 13, 17, 43, 65–68, 70, 72, 73, 83–85, 111–119, 134, 139, 141, 144, 147, 185, 186
brainstorm, 61
branch, 166
break, 26, 169
breath, 34, 50
breathing, 49, 50, 55, 67, 73, 78, 80, 86, 87, 90, 107
brew, 131
buffer, 93, 95, 99, 185
building, 59, 95, 97–99, 101, 175, 176, 183, 184
bullying, 145
burden, 11, 159, 164
burnout, 7, 101, 104

cactus, 131
caffeine, 86
calm, 49, 55, 80, 90
campaign, 178
capacity, 84
car, 82
care, 5, 7, 9–11, 13–16, 18–21, 24, 36, 54, 59, 67, 74, 92, 94, 96, 101–109, 119–124,

128, 130, 131, 135, 136,
138, 145, 148–150, 152,
153, 157–159, 161–180,
183–191
career, 41
Carl Rogers, 4
case, 47, 75, 140, 141, 147, 155
catalyst, 135, 185
catharsis, 57, 58
cause, 89, 99
caution, 59
cell, 112
censorship, 60
century, 4, 5, 29, 42
challenge, 9, 10, 13, 17, 24–27, 33,
39, 45, 56, 76, 98, 100,
107, 108, 163, 167, 173,
178
change, 27, 41, 133, 175–178, 183,
184, 187
chatter, 49
chemical, 13, 14, 112, 143
chemistry, 17
childcare, 169
childhood, 4
choice, 45
chore, 81
circulation, 82
clarity, 49, 55, 56, 61, 73, 82, 185
class, 74, 82
classification, 4, 134
clay, 45
client, 23, 24, 28, 43
clock, 85, 88, 89
club, 80
co, 24
cognition, 66, 70, 112
coherence, 57

collaboration, 2, 13, 14, 16, 22, 36,
69, 119, 124, 130, 135,
136, 148–150, 156, 159,
161, 169, 179, 181–184,
187–189, 191
collaborative, 13, 18, 23, 28, 163,
164, 179
collage, 39, 42, 46
collection, 130, 154, 180
color, 151
combat, 9, 75, 97, 161
combination, 16, 17, 26, 28, 42, 46,
49, 75, 80, 128, 140, 147,
167
comfort, 75, 96, 98, 169
commitment, 13, 24, 32, 56, 81, 83,
148, 184
communication, 6, 44, 46, 66, 68,
94, 96, 98, 99, 118, 130,
163, 164, 169, 176, 178
community, 2, 5, 9, 15, 18, 19, 21,
40, 42, 46, 82, 94–98, 100,
130, 135, 159–161, 163,
172–176, 178–182, 184,
185, 188
companionship, 99
compassion, 31, 36, 59, 61,
105–107, 173, 185
compatibility, 128
competence, 15, 16, 20, 21, 127,
148–150, 154
competency, 149, 161
complement, 19, 69, 133, 173, 174
complexity, 14, 18, 113, 117, 119,
139, 143, 167
compliance, 93
component, 14, 17, 24, 50, 74, 76,
164, 179, 185
composition, 66

compound, 175
compulsion, 26
concentration, 7, 43, 49, 50, 80, 84, 85, 88
concept, 16, 20, 52, 60, 143, 146, 150, 165
concern, 62, 132
conclusion, 15, 16, 27, 31, 48, 56, 63, 67, 89, 100, 104, 108, 116, 128, 131, 133, 138, 140, 171, 181, 187, 188
condition, 9, 33, 75, 84, 146, 172
conductance, 129
conferencing, 169
confidence, 75, 80, 175
confidentiality, 130, 170, 177
confinement, 4
conjunction, 27
connectedness, 15, 99, 188
connection, 5, 15, 16, 51–54, 65, 67, 68, 75, 80, 93, 94, 97, 111, 119, 143, 172, 185, 186
connectivity, 114, 116, 169
consciousness, 43
consent, 128, 135–138, 147, 172, 177
consideration, 15, 147, 186
consistency, 56, 74
consolidation, 84
consultation, 149, 163
consumption, 69
contact, 162
contamination, 26
context, 5, 8, 14, 16, 19, 21, 22, 119, 120, 150, 151, 153, 154, 169, 181
continuity, 124, 164, 171
contrast, 20

control, 63, 75, 112, 114, 117, 143, 181
controversy, 131, 133
convenience, 124, 129
convergence, 165
coordination, 19, 163, 164
coping, 18, 24, 25, 28, 58, 59, 61, 93, 94, 100, 129, 183, 184, 188
cord, 111
core, 23, 27, 35, 49, 52, 112
cornerstone, 114
cortex, 112, 117
cortisol, 49, 73
cost, 11, 116, 147, 159, 170
counseling, 42, 120, 173
counselor, 97
counterculture, 132
country, 178
coverage, 11, 167, 177, 178
creation, 185, 188
creativity, 41, 45, 58
criminalization, 132
crisis, 10–13
culture, 9, 21, 22, 108, 149, 150, 186, 190
curiosity, 149
curricula, 21
cycle, 12, 26, 85, 89
cycling, 73, 77

dance, 39
dancing, 73, 77
Daniel Goleman, 56
data, 128–130, 146, 147, 154, 170–172, 180, 181
day, 51, 74, 81, 83, 86, 89, 107, 129
daytime, 87–89
decision, 7, 84, 85, 112, 137, 163, 164, 176, 180–182

decline, 68, 73, 131
decriminalization, 133
dedication, 56
deficiency, 68, 69
definition, 2, 120
Deinstitutionalization, 5
deinstitutionalization, 5
delivery, 120, 124, 148, 164, 169, 172, 189
demand, 120, 163
denial, 8
departure, 184
depression, 6, 7, 18, 25, 33, 43, 55, 58, 61, 63, 65, 66, 68, 70, 73–76, 80, 84, 85, 87, 88, 93, 96, 99, 113, 115, 117, 118, 133, 139–143, 147, 148, 155, 156, 184–186
deprivation, 83–85, 87, 88
design, 154, 156
destigmatization, 2, 5
destination, 82
detachment, 7
determinant, 7
determination, 173, 192
detoxification, 50
devaluation, 8
development, 4, 6, 21, 25, 68, 69, 84, 85, 87, 88, 100, 113, 118, 119, 123, 128, 131, 140, 141, 144, 145, 155, 156, 160, 166, 169, 173, 176, 180, 182, 183, 187, 188
device, 128, 172
diabetes, 2, 85
diagnosis, 4, 13, 120
diet, 66, 67, 69, 70, 72, 139, 143, 185
difficulty, 25, 28, 56, 87, 127

diffusion, 116
digestion, 111
dignity, 4, 114
dimension, 15
dinner, 81
disability, 151, 160
disadvantage, 12
discipline, 42, 49
disclosure, 63, 99
discomfort, 35, 88, 127
discontinuation, 81
discourse, 132
discovery, 41, 60, 185
discrimination, 2, 7–11, 100, 118, 151, 160, 161, 163, 173, 175, 176, 180, 183, 187, 188
disease, 2, 6, 73
disorder, 25, 26, 35, 84–87, 116, 140, 166, 172, 174
distance, 44, 82
distortion, 25
distress, 6, 61, 63, 99, 136, 160, 185
diversity, 9, 20, 45, 67, 98, 100, 120, 149, 156
divide, 119
doorknob, 26
dopamine, 43, 66, 68, 73, 84, 87
doubt, 48
drain, 11
drawing, 39, 42, 46
drug, 34, 166, 168
duration, 56, 57, 74, 76, 81, 85, 129
dynamic, 2, 41, 50, 94, 139, 145
dysbiosis, 118
dysfunction, 66

ear, 97
ease, 157

eating, 26, 68, 69, 183
edge, 184, 187, 189
educating, 92
education, 2, 9, 21, 95, 98, 149, 150, 153, 160, 163, 164, 174, 176, 179, 181, 182, 184
effect, 73, 74, 178
effectiveness, 18, 19, 24, 28, 42, 45–48, 58, 62, 63, 70, 106, 127, 128, 130, 133, 145, 147, 148, 150, 156, 170, 171, 177, 180, 182, 186, 189, 190
efficacy, 8, 69, 133, 147, 166, 188
efficiency, 128, 129, 180
effort, 13, 18, 93, 94, 96, 99
electronic, 86, 90, 120
electrophysiology, 113
elevator, 74, 82
emergence, 3, 4
Emil Kraepelin, 4
emotion, 45, 141
empathy, 9, 92, 94, 96–100, 173, 176
emphasis, 23, 50
employment, 9, 160, 179, 180, 182
empowerment, 45, 57, 63, 164, 182, 188
encouragement, 92, 100, 173, 174
end, 45
endeavor, 114
endocrine, 66
endurance, 50, 77
energy, 68, 75, 93
engagement, 17, 23, 37, 75, 93, 97, 98, 127, 130, 148, 150, 161, 164, 170, 173, 178, 182, 184
entry, 76

environment, 9, 29, 35, 38, 45, 61, 85, 90, 92, 98, 100, 126, 127, 139, 143–145, 160, 163, 170, 178, 180, 181, 186
epigenetic, 139–143, 145
equality, 10
equine, 19
equipment, 116, 128, 170
equity, 120, 135, 147, 153, 157–159, 178, 186
error, 92
establishment, 4, 182
esteem, 1, 8, 47, 61, 74, 75, 80, 93, 95, 96, 98–100, 185
ethnicity, 154, 160, 179
evaluation, 18, 21, 86, 93, 177, 178
evening, 81, 86
event, 27
evidence, 14, 18, 21, 24, 27, 29, 36, 42, 47, 52, 58, 67, 69, 75, 131, 135, 147, 163, 172, 176–178, 180, 189
evil, 3
exacerbation, 8, 144
example, 2, 17–20, 25–27, 47, 66, 81, 82, 94, 107, 112, 116–118, 131, 133, 139, 143, 146, 151, 154, 155, 159, 166, 167, 174, 179, 183, 185
exception, 169
excess, 69
exchange, 94
exclusion, 2, 8, 145, 160, 180
exercise, 15, 45, 49, 59, 67, 73–77, 79–83, 86, 185
exhibit, 117
exorcism, 3, 4

expense, 108
experience, 2, 6–9, 11, 24, 34, 41, 45, 51, 55, 59, 76, 79, 87, 96, 99, 118, 127, 128, 135–137, 151, 154, 162, 174, 176–178, 181, 182
experiment, 83
expertise, 18, 45, 116, 128, 137, 149, 170, 176
exploration, 28, 39, 45, 57, 126, 133, 145, 167, 184–186
exposure, 23–26, 86, 90, 118, 126–128, 143, 171
expression, 19, 39, 41, 42, 46, 47, 57, 60, 62, 92, 113, 138–145, 150, 186
extent, 163
eye, 85

face, 28, 56, 100, 107, 120, 130, 151, 157, 159, 162, 163
factor, 99, 118, 133, 144
failure, 14, 167
family, 17–19, 96, 107, 108, 150
father, 4
fatigue, 68, 75, 87, 88
fatty, 69, 70, 72, 143
fear, 9, 26, 48, 113, 173, 188
fee, 161
feedback, 93, 127, 128, 130, 171
feeling, 55, 75, 107
fiber, 66, 112
field, 2, 5, 13–15, 21, 41, 42, 48, 67, 111, 114, 116, 117, 119, 120, 128, 131, 133, 135, 137–139, 145–147, 153, 165–167, 169, 172, 175, 176, 178, 186, 187, 189, 190

finding, 50, 81, 83, 109
fish, 68, 69, 143
fitness, 50, 51, 74, 80–82, 129, 170, 185
flexibility, 49, 50, 55
flourishing, 187
flow, 43, 57, 73
flying, 126
focus, 4, 9, 13, 16, 23, 26, 35, 39, 45, 49, 51, 55, 58, 61, 74, 104, 139, 147, 161, 163, 179, 180
folate, 68
follow, 75, 128
following, 45, 47, 48, 104, 134, 156, 190, 191
food, 26, 69, 70
force, 32
forefront, 172
form, 6, 42, 44, 46, 57, 61–63, 81, 92, 185
formation, 100, 134, 139
formulation, 23
Foster, 69, 94, 96, 100
foster, 6, 10, 19, 21, 42, 48, 54, 58, 59, 93, 97, 100, 130, 131, 150, 173, 178, 182, 187, 188, 190
fostering, 2, 9, 14, 43, 57, 62, 92, 95, 96, 98, 100, 156, 159, 163, 175, 177, 178, 182, 185, 187, 188, 191
foundation, 4, 96, 106, 185
fragmentation, 162
framework, 5, 19, 57, 100, 137, 138, 151
Freewriting, 57
freewriting, 57
friend, 74

frustration, 81, 88, 89
fulfillment, 5, 7, 183
fullness, 69
fun, 74
function, 2, 6, 13, 55, 58, 65–68, 70, 72, 73, 76, 80, 83–85, 113–116, 118, 139, 141, 143, 185
functioning, 11, 58, 87–89, 144, 185
fundamental, 2, 54, 87, 104, 105, 107, 179, 184
funding, 5, 8, 174, 176, 179, 180, 183
future, 13, 15, 18, 36, 67, 83, 98, 114, 116, 120, 123, 124, 128, 129, 131, 136, 145, 162, 165, 167, 169, 171, 178, 181, 184, 186, 187

Galen, 3
gap, 163, 179
gardening, 79
gear, 83
gender, 1, 151, 154, 160
Gene, 143
gene, 113, 138–145, 166, 186
genetic, 13, 139–142, 145–147, 165–168, 186, 187
genomic, 140
gestalt, 39
go, 45, 55, 162
goal, 23, 25, 45, 76, 81, 166
government, 132
grammar, 62
gratitude, 58, 97
green, 160
greenery, 80
grief, 59
grounding, 59, 177

group, 1, 8, 21, 74, 80–82, 94, 97, 100, 139, 150, 154, 174, 175, 178
growth, 4, 39, 41, 42, 44, 45, 48, 55, 57–62, 66, 98, 108, 173
guarantee, 167
guidance, 18, 35, 59, 62, 63, 75, 92, 96, 97, 106, 108, 130, 171, 173, 174, 182
guilt, 8, 25, 107, 108
gut, 65–67, 118, 119, 185

habit, 80, 81, 83
hallmark, 84
halt, 132
hand, 8, 23, 55, 68, 84, 96, 97, 99, 120
handling, 59
handwashing, 26
happiness, 58, 73, 185
harm, 128, 137
harmony, 49
healing, 18, 39, 41, 42, 45, 52, 57, 59, 60, 131, 134, 150, 185
health, 1–22, 24–34, 36, 38, 40–42, 44–49, 51–60, 62, 63, 65–80, 83–87, 89, 92–101, 108, 111–114, 116–124, 126, 128–154, 156–191
healthcare, 2, 9, 11, 13, 18, 19, 29, 74–76, 86, 91, 117, 118, 120, 128–131, 160, 162–165, 167, 176, 179, 182, 187, 188
heart, 6, 73, 77, 129, 170, 191
heartbeat, 111
heat, 50

help, 7, 8, 11, 15, 17–20, 23, 25, 33–35, 39, 55–57, 62, 63, 66, 67, 69, 70, 74, 75, 79–82, 86, 89–100, 102, 105, 106, 114, 116, 127, 129, 143, 146, 149–151, 154, 156, 160, 161, 163, 164, 169, 171, 174–176, 181, 187, 188
helpline, 95
heterogeneity, 146
hiking, 74, 79–81
histone, 139, 140
history, 3, 33, 59, 131, 133, 134
home, 51, 65, 75, 85
homelessness, 5, 11
homophobia, 20
honor, 45, 97
hope, 59, 114, 173, 174, 182
hopelessness, 33, 75
hormone, 55, 89, 112
hour, 82, 86, 90
housing, 9, 160, 180, 182
humanism, 4
humility, 21, 149
Humphry Osmond, 132
hunger, 69
hygiene, 85, 129, 185
hyperactivity, 35
hypertension, 6
hypothalamus, 112
hypothesis, 57

idea, 97
identification, 179
identity, 58, 151
illness, 1, 5, 6, 8, 10, 11, 13, 19, 85, 176, 180
image, 26, 61, 74, 116

imagery, 90
imaging, 115, 116
imbalance, 87
immersion, 127
impact, 2, 4–8, 10, 11, 14, 15, 17, 18, 20, 34, 52, 55, 66, 67, 70, 71, 73, 75, 76, 85, 87, 89, 90, 93, 97–99, 113, 118, 119, 129, 139, 144, 147, 151, 154, 160, 166, 172, 176–178, 180, 184–187
impairment, 68
impatience, 56
implementation, 121, 122, 124, 148, 159, 180
importance, 2–5, 14–17, 21, 23, 39, 49, 57, 66, 68, 74, 95, 96, 98, 108, 114, 117, 118, 136, 148, 149, 151, 155, 159, 162, 175, 177–179, 184, 185, 188, 189
improve, 5, 27, 30, 35, 48, 49, 51, 55, 56, 67, 70, 73–76, 79–83, 85, 89–92, 119, 127, 133, 136, 145, 146, 158, 164, 166–169, 178, 180, 183, 188, 190, 191
improvement, 18, 177, 178
improving, 31, 35, 54, 55, 63, 67, 72, 74, 89, 90, 114, 120, 124, 128, 148, 159, 162, 163, 165, 170, 172, 181, 183, 189
impulsivity, 35
in, 2–9, 11, 13–21, 23–30, 32–43, 45–52, 54–63, 65–77, 79–90, 92–101, 104, 106–108, 112–121, 123,

Index

124, 126–151, 153–191
inattention, 35
incarceration, 11
incense, 51
inclusion, 100, 120, 149, 180, 188
inclusivity, 9, 10, 45, 98, 161
income, 11, 159, 160, 179
increase, 6, 49–51, 60, 73, 74, 77, 80–82, 84, 85, 113, 128, 144, 148, 149, 153, 160, 169, 186, 190
India, 49
individual, 2, 4, 8, 11, 14–18, 21, 24, 26, 27, 29, 35, 38, 46, 49, 59, 63, 69, 71, 75, 81, 83, 92, 97, 99, 100, 108, 117–119, 127, 128, 130, 139, 145–151, 161, 165, 166, 168–170, 175, 177, 178, 185–187
individualization, 43
indulgence, 107
inequality, 160
inflammation, 6, 49, 66, 143, 144
influence, 2, 7, 17, 19, 21, 22, 65, 66, 70, 73, 85, 97, 118, 139, 140, 142–144, 148, 151, 152, 154, 160, 185, 186, 188
information, 92, 94, 95, 100, 107, 114, 119, 127, 129, 130, 137, 142, 143, 146, 147, 164, 166, 168, 170, 171, 177, 181
infrastructure, 147
initiative, 159
injury, 115
innovation, 2, 13, 119, 124, 131, 187, 189–191

input, 18
insight, 3, 4, 57, 62, 63, 104, 113, 173
insomnia, 55, 84, 87, 90
instance, 6, 26, 113, 147, 169, 179, 184
institutionalization, 5
instructor, 51
insurance, 11, 167, 178
intake, 69, 70, 77, 86
integration, 5, 7, 9, 16, 36, 41, 48, 57, 97, 99, 116, 119, 123, 128, 130, 131, 135, 136, 138, 161–166, 170, 179, 180, 186, 188, 189
integrity, 66, 116
intelligence, 114, 128, 187
intensity, 58, 59, 74, 76, 81, 171
intention, 45
intentionality, 93, 96
interaction, 19
interconnectedness, 2, 11, 15, 17, 19, 20, 165, 184
interconnection, 52
interest, 4, 25, 33, 94, 132–135, 138
internalization, 8
internet, 169
interplay, 2, 3, 5, 14, 141–143, 145, 186, 188
interpretation, 19, 116
intersectionality, 151, 153, 161, 186
intervention, 10, 21, 29, 31, 34, 42, 62, 63, 117, 119, 135, 136, 139, 155, 156, 159, 166, 179–181, 183, 187, 188
introspection, 4, 49, 135
investing, 90, 98
investment, 94, 107, 131

involve, 9, 18, 20, 23–26, 50, 55, 94, 97, 107, 108, 147, 150, 161, 167, 183
involvement, 18, 19, 97, 131, 141, 148, 164, 180, 182
iron, 69
irritability, 87, 89
isolation, 7, 8, 11, 15, 74, 93, 96, 97, 130, 144, 160, 173, 182, 187
issue, 9, 10, 159, 162, 178

job, 7, 79, 85, 160
John J. Ratey, 75
journal, 59, 76, 82
journaling, 60, 61, 86
journey, 13, 14, 41, 48, 51, 56, 60, 62, 83, 106, 108, 169, 171, 173–175, 184, 186
joy, 7, 58, 80, 81, 83
judgment, 29, 35, 50, 60, 90, 94, 163, 185, 188
justice, 5, 153

key, 3, 6, 7, 12, 15, 16, 28, 30, 39, 43, 47, 49, 51, 52, 55, 57, 58, 65–68, 70, 81, 90, 93, 99, 101, 109, 117, 120, 129, 139, 141, 143, 146, 148, 152, 154, 162, 166, 169, 172, 176, 178, 180, 187
kindness, 105
knowledge, 2, 41, 92, 96, 107, 108, 113, 114, 139, 140, 145, 147, 149, 163, 176, 179, 181, 189

lack, 5, 8, 11, 28, 88, 96, 107, 108, 159, 163
lamb, 68
landscape, 13, 22, 57, 98, 131, 136, 138, 156, 161, 165, 169, 175, 181, 183, 184, 186–189, 191
language, 21, 44, 154
layer, 112
lead, 7–9, 11, 14, 49, 57, 58, 68, 81, 85–89, 130, 131, 145, 150, 160, 162, 184, 187, 188, 190
learn, 24–26, 48, 51, 149, 182
learning, 5, 41, 48, 75, 84, 108, 116, 146
legalization, 133
legislation, 178
length, 56
lens, 151
level, 2, 11, 50, 80, 81, 127, 175, 183
leverage, 169, 172
lie, 60, 186, 187, 192
life, 1, 6, 7, 9, 11, 15, 16, 18, 24, 28, 31, 49, 51, 54–57, 59, 72–76, 81–83, 88, 89, 92, 96–98, 104, 106, 107, 113, 127, 144, 162, 185, 186
lifespan, 6
lifestyle, 15, 49, 56, 76, 82, 90, 92, 129, 130, 147, 165–167, 171
lifetime, 139
light, 82, 86, 90, 113, 114, 142, 187
likelihood, 74, 148, 166, 167
limit, 90, 159, 163
limitation, 14, 28
link, 67, 69, 70
listening, 92, 94–97, 99
literacy, 163, 179–181
literature, 172
living, 8, 15, 49, 114, 169

lobbying, 177
lobe, 112
location, 13, 179
loneliness, 15, 96, 97, 173
longevity, 6
loss, 25, 33, 43, 59
love, 92, 99, 107
lunch, 107
luxury, 104

machine, 90, 116, 146
magnesium, 68–70, 72
mainstream, 128, 135, 138, 186
maintenance, 28
makeup, 4, 145, 165, 166, 186
making, 6, 7, 39, 42–45, 50, 57, 58, 70, 76, 80, 82, 84, 85, 112, 163, 164, 180–182, 188
management, 16, 24, 86, 90, 120, 127–130, 164, 174, 183, 187
manifestation, 113
manner, 33, 39, 56, 96, 185
marginalization, 8, 11, 160
Maria, 79, 80
marketing, 79
material, 166
matter, 83, 115, 116
MBCT, 33
meaning, 7, 14, 15, 57, 137
means, 42, 46, 47, 49, 60, 120, 169
measure, 18, 129, 177
measurement, 19
meat, 68, 69
mechanism, 63, 73, 139
medication, 11, 14, 17, 18, 24, 28, 47, 69, 93, 94, 146, 147, 166, 167
medicine, 146, 165–169, 187

meditation, 15, 29, 33, 34, 48–51, 54–56, 67, 86, 90, 107, 171
Mediterranean, 72, 143
melatonin, 89, 90
member, 175
memory, 7, 58, 73, 84, 85, 112, 139
mentoring, 173, 174
mentorship, 149, 182
message, 177, 178
messaging, 120, 130, 176, 178
messenger, 139
meta, 58
metabolism, 68, 166
methyl, 139
methylation, 139, 140
microbiota, 65–67, 118
mind, 4, 15–17, 39, 49–56, 59, 74, 76, 78–80, 90, 149, 171, 184, 186
mindedness, 149
mindfulness, 14, 15, 29, 31–38, 43, 49, 54–56, 59, 66, 69, 74, 75, 78, 80, 86, 90, 101, 107, 183, 185
mindset, 55, 101, 149
mineral, 68
misalignment, 88
mistreatment, 3
misuse, 135
mobile, 75, 108, 120, 188
mobilization, 176
modality, 28, 39, 42
model, 3–5, 13–17, 19, 20, 95, 163
modification, 139
molecule, 139
moment, 33–35, 43, 45, 55, 90, 185
momentum, 82, 165

monitoring, 26, 114, 120, 128–131, 170, 171, 186
mood, 13, 18, 43, 55, 61, 66–68, 70–76, 80, 84, 85, 87, 88, 107, 134, 141, 171, 174, 185
morning, 75, 81
mortality, 6
motility, 66
motion, 128
motivation, 7, 17, 24, 80–83, 89, 108, 170
motor, 82, 112
movement, 5, 34, 49, 50, 55, 74, 80, 132, 137
muscle, 77, 90
music, 39

narcolepsy, 89
narrative, 57, 59
nature, 8, 10, 13, 17, 18, 20, 28, 41, 44, 54, 74, 79, 80, 89, 96, 99, 101, 117, 137, 139, 142, 150, 178, 184, 186
necessity, 104
need, 5, 9, 14–16, 45, 92, 94, 97, 99, 104, 107, 119, 122, 130, 133, 135, 137, 147, 156, 157, 159, 161–163, 167, 169, 170, 181, 184
neighboring, 112
nerve, 66
network, 7, 18, 66, 99, 100
neuroimaging, 113, 114, 116, 117, 119, 146, 186
neuroinflammation, 66
neuron, 112
neuroplasticity, 134, 141
neuroscience, 2, 113, 114

neurotransmitter, 66, 68, 70, 140, 143, 147
nicotine, 86
night, 86, 87
noise, 85, 90, 160
non, 33, 38, 39, 44, 61, 63, 87, 132, 139, 163, 173
nourishment, 101
novel, 67, 118, 131, 133, 136, 141, 142, 190
nucleus, 112
number, 93
nurture, 98, 100, 101
nutrient, 68–70, 72
nutrition, 15, 66–70, 185
nutritionist, 18

obesity, 85
object, 50
observation, 178
obsession, 26
occipital, 112
offer, 7, 18, 30, 37, 48, 51, 55, 56, 67, 75, 76, 94, 98–100, 117, 127, 129, 171, 173, 174, 184
oil, 143
one, 15, 17, 20, 24, 35, 51, 57, 59, 60, 62, 63, 68, 74, 76, 79, 83, 84, 87, 95, 101, 107, 108, 112, 145, 149, 165, 168, 172, 185
onset, 70, 85
opinion, 133, 176
opportunity, 94
oppression, 20, 151
optimism, 132
option, 133
order, 15, 89, 112, 189

organ, 112
organization, 159
other, 2, 6, 8, 14, 15, 18, 20, 23, 24, 26–29, 36, 39, 41, 42, 46, 47, 55, 66, 68–70, 73, 78, 81, 84, 96, 97, 99, 100, 108, 112, 116, 120, 128, 151, 163, 165, 167, 168, 174, 176, 182, 186
outcome, 61
outlet, 57, 62, 63
outlook, 55
outreach, 159, 163
overemphasis, 14
overview, 10, 130
overwhelm, 74
ownership, 182
oxygen, 68, 77

pain, 49, 55, 127, 128
painting, 39, 42, 46, 48
pair, 174
panacea, 43, 167
paper, 45, 62, 185
Paracelsus, 4
paradigm, 5, 168
parallel, 138
parity, 178
part, 15, 49, 68, 70, 74, 79, 81–83, 94, 97, 98, 108, 167, 169
participation, 23, 37, 93, 182
partner, 82
partnership, 21
past, 5
pathogenesis, 66
pathway, 66
patience, 55, 56, 83
patient, 92, 106, 135, 137, 146, 149, 150, 162, 166, 172

pattern, 25
peace, 15, 29, 49, 51
peer, 130, 173–175, 182, 184, 188
pen, 185
people, 1, 8, 49, 55, 89, 94, 100, 154, 181
perception, 8, 19, 107, 112, 127, 148
performance, 7, 26, 83–85, 89, 185
period, 4
persecution, 4
persistence, 160
person, 1, 14–19, 25–27, 39, 83, 95, 96, 101, 130, 145, 149, 151, 167, 169, 189, 191
perspective, 4, 25, 57–59, 63, 93, 119, 142, 184, 186
peyote, 131
phenomenon, 11
philosophy, 49
phone, 120, 169
phosphorylation, 139
physician, 3, 4
place, 59, 106, 130, 137
plan, 23, 28, 44, 47, 75, 105, 106, 166, 167, 174, 178
planning, 28, 81, 114, 182
plasticity, 68, 139, 143
pleasure, 25, 43, 73
poetry, 39
point, 80, 81, 87, 118, 162
policy, 9, 10, 137, 153, 161, 164, 176, 178–181, 183, 184, 187
pollution, 160
popularity, 55, 129, 131
population, 87, 154, 172, 175, 181
portion, 175
portrayal, 8, 132
pose, 108

position, 50
positivity, 106
possession, 3, 20
posture, 49, 55
potential, 10, 17, 35, 55, 67, 70, 83, 114, 117–119, 123, 124, 126, 128–138, 140–142, 145, 148, 155, 162, 167, 168, 171, 172, 174, 178, 183, 186–188
poultry, 68, 69
poverty, 11, 118, 180
power, 20, 41, 45, 51, 53, 57, 60, 67, 83, 98, 100, 175, 177
practice, 18, 24, 28, 29, 32, 36–39, 45, 48–51, 55, 56, 58, 60–62, 90, 101, 107, 126–128, 140, 142, 147, 153, 169, 172, 185–187
practitioner, 51
precision, 146, 171
predisposition, 147, 166
presence, 24, 97, 98, 127
presentation, 117
preservation, 107
pressure, 6, 55, 58
prevalence, 9–11, 13, 162, 180
prevention, 1, 145, 179–181, 183, 187
primary, 49, 161–164, 167, 180, 187, 188
principle, 136
prioritize, 2, 9, 16, 19, 69, 74, 85, 89, 98, 101, 104, 107, 108, 161, 179, 180, 183, 185, 187
priority, 76, 81, 83
privacy, 114, 128, 130, 147, 167, 169, 172, 177

problem, 7, 24, 58, 73
process, 5, 8, 13, 17, 18, 23, 26, 28, 39, 41–43, 45, 48, 56–63, 83, 94, 106, 109, 126, 139, 143, 145, 148, 149, 184, 185
processing, 19, 48, 59, 62, 112, 113, 134, 145
product, 45, 143
production, 66, 68, 73, 89, 90, 112
productivity, 5, 7, 11, 85
professional, 21, 41, 58, 59, 74–76, 79, 86, 91, 92, 97, 135, 137, 159, 171, 172, 174
proficiency, 169
profile, 135, 146, 166
prognosis, 146
program, 54, 159, 172
progress, 51, 76, 82, 83, 114, 128, 171, 177
progression, 6, 70, 85, 140, 166
prominence, 5
promise, 30, 35, 61, 63, 114, 116, 118, 122, 127, 133, 136, 142, 147, 148, 167, 169, 186–188
promotion, 1, 2, 180, 183
proposal, 172
protection, 68
protein, 143
provider, 75, 91
provision, 21, 92, 93, 172, 180
psilocybin, 133, 186
psychedelic, 131–133, 135–138
psychiatrist, 18
psychiatry, 4, 111, 132
psychoanalysis, 4
psychoeducation, 24, 129
psychology, 2, 3, 29, 31, 41

psychotherapy, 18, 69, 133, 135, 147, 167
public, 8, 26, 126, 132, 133, 163, 176, 179, 181, 183
pumpkin, 68
punctuation, 62
purpose, 7, 15, 97, 137, 183

qigong, 74
quality, 5, 6, 9, 11, 18, 55, 58, 61, 72, 73, 75, 76, 80, 83–93, 95, 99, 127–129, 161, 162, 169, 175, 177, 182, 183, 188, 189
quo, 178

race, 20, 151, 154, 160
racism, 20
radiation, 115
rainforest, 131
range, 2, 14, 24, 40, 44, 46, 48, 79, 85, 101, 121, 129, 139, 171, 174
rapport, 28, 119
rate, 6, 73, 77, 129, 170
reach, 94, 99, 186
reaction, 84
readiness, 62, 63
reading, 86, 90, 108
reality, 116, 126, 127, 171, 172, 186
realization, 49, 186
realm, 3, 126, 183
reassurance, 92
recognition, 5, 14, 15, 29, 49, 67, 117, 118, 132, 133, 137, 151
record, 120
recovery, 5, 9, 10, 14, 93, 173–175, 188

reduction, 18, 43, 49, 50, 59, 63, 66, 73–75, 80, 107, 179, 180, 187
referral, 163, 164
reflection, 21, 28, 45, 49, 59–62, 149
region, 117
regulation, 6, 19, 31, 35, 57, 58, 66, 80, 84, 87, 88, 117, 134, 135, 139, 141, 144, 145, 185
rehabilitation, 1, 46
reimbursement, 164
relapse, 33
relation, 151
relationship, 23, 28, 39, 51, 54, 68, 84, 96, 97
relaxation, 17, 24, 34, 43, 49, 50, 55, 56, 59, 74, 78, 86, 90, 101, 183
release, 57, 58, 60, 73, 135
reliability, 97, 130, 171
reliance, 14
relief, 14, 185
religion, 154
reluctance, 188
reminder, 81
replacement, 44, 69
representation, 153
representative, 177
rescheduling, 137
research, 2, 5, 18, 19, 21, 22, 36, 52, 63, 67, 70, 73, 113, 114, 116–119, 124, 128, 131–137, 139–143, 145–148, 153–156, 162, 167, 169, 170, 177, 180, 184, 186, 187, 189–191
resilience, 1, 7, 9, 15, 31, 34, 36, 48, 54, 57–59, 80, 93, 95, 98,

100, 101, 104, 106, 107, 119, 144, 150, 182–184, 188
resistance, 77
resource, 161, 164, 169, 176, 180
respect, 45, 51, 56, 94, 99, 150, 154, 173, 177
response, 43, 55, 68, 87, 117, 129, 139–141, 146, 147, 166, 179
responsibility, 9, 182
responsiveness, 144, 166
rest, 83
restlessness, 88
restoration, 87
restructuring, 24–26, 60, 63
result, 11, 76, 88, 89, 132, 137, 167, 177
resurgence, 132, 134
review, 137, 172
revival, 131–133
reward, 43
rhythm, 89
riding, 19
right, 45
rise, 5, 146
risk, 2, 11, 68, 70–73, 84, 85, 87, 93, 96, 99, 113, 137, 139, 143, 144, 160, 166, 167, 179, 180
role, 4–9, 14, 15, 17, 19, 22, 28, 39, 42, 45, 51, 65–72, 76, 83, 85, 87, 89, 90, 92, 93, 95, 96, 98–101, 112, 118, 129, 131, 137–140, 143, 145, 148, 153, 160, 162, 164, 166, 172, 174, 175, 181, 183, 185–187, 189
room, 50

root, 13, 16, 119
routine, 50, 55, 74–76, 79–83, 86, 89, 92, 102, 104–106, 167, 169, 170
run, 174
running, 73, 77, 80

sadness, 25, 33, 75
safeguard, 130, 137
safety, 59, 132, 133, 135, 137, 166, 186
Sarah, 47, 48, 54, 75, 94, 174, 175
satisfaction, 7, 58, 81, 83, 96, 98, 150, 185
scale, 147, 161
scan, 34
schedule, 56, 81, 85, 88, 89
schizophrenia, 85, 115, 116, 139, 142, 166
school, 178
sclerosis, 115
scope, 1, 2, 120
screening, 135, 164, 180
sculpture, 39, 42, 46
secretion, 66
section, 3, 5, 10, 42, 46, 49, 51, 55, 60, 67, 70, 73, 76, 80, 83, 87, 89, 92, 96, 98, 104, 106, 107, 114, 117, 120, 126, 129, 131, 136, 143, 145, 148, 157, 160, 162, 169, 173, 175, 178, 181, 189
security, 92, 93, 99, 130, 170–172
selection, 147, 148
self, 1, 4, 8, 21, 26, 28, 29, 31, 35, 36, 39, 41–51, 55, 57–62, 74, 75, 80, 93, 95, 96, 98–109, 128, 134, 149,

150, 164, 170, 171, 173,
    185, 186, 188
sense, 6, 7, 15, 29, 48, 49, 55, 57–59,
    61, 63, 75, 80, 82, 83,
    92–100, 127, 130,
    173–175, 177, 182, 183,
    185, 188
sensitivity, 45, 56
sensor, 171
sequence, 50, 138, 143, 166
series, 50
service, 174, 180
session, 57
setting, 57, 81, 83, 107, 108, 135,
    186
severity, 85
sexism, 20
sexuality, 151, 160
shame, 8
shape, 15, 19, 26, 36, 114, 118, 124,
    136, 145, 150, 154, 156,
    160, 165, 181, 184, 187,
    189, 191
share, 18, 82, 94, 100, 173, 176, 182
sharing, 96, 97, 130, 161, 171, 173,
    175, 177
shift, 3–5, 15, 16, 118, 168, 187
shortage, 11, 163
sickness, 128
side, 133, 166, 167
Sigmund Freud, 4, 39
sign, 154
significance, 51, 57, 83, 92, 95, 100,
    136, 173, 184
size, 24, 51, 95, 145, 149, 165, 168
skill, 24, 45, 56
skin, 129
sleep, 15, 25, 55, 58, 68, 73, 75, 80,
    83–92, 129, 170, 185

sleepiness, 87, 89
smartphone, 128, 129, 146
snack, 83
socializing, 99
society, 2, 3, 101, 150, 155, 156, 173,
    175, 178, 187
socio, 17, 151
sociology, 2
solace, 59
solidarity, 177
solitude, 97
solution, 120, 145, 165
solving, 7, 24, 58, 73
source, 94
space, 42, 45, 49, 51, 94, 96, 97, 99,
    173, 182
span, 84
speaking, 26, 96, 126
specialist, 91
specialty, 4
spectrum, 65, 118, 127
spelling, 62
spinach, 68, 69
spirit, 49, 184, 186
spirituality, 15
stability, 83, 99, 160, 161
standard, 69, 123
Stanislav Grof, 132
start, 51, 75, 81, 108
starting, 26, 74, 76, 81
state, 6, 10, 43, 49, 50, 55
status, 10, 13, 17, 130, 151, 154,
    160, 178
step, 72, 104, 162, 181
stigma, 7–11, 13, 14, 98, 100, 151,
    154, 162–164, 169, 173,
    175, 176, 178–181, 183,
    184, 187, 188, 191
stigmatization, 3

stimulation, 148
stimulus, 171
storage, 130
story, 57
strain, 11
strategy, 81, 82, 181–183
street, 94
strength, 49, 50, 55, 74, 76, 77, 79, 80
stress, 1, 6, 7, 34, 43, 49–51, 54–56, 59, 63, 66–68, 73, 74, 76, 79, 80, 86–90, 92, 93, 95, 96, 98–101, 104, 107, 129, 139–141, 143–145, 151, 160, 183, 185
stretching, 55, 74, 82
structure, 13, 28, 113, 114, 116, 138
struggle, 28, 35, 55, 61, 88, 89, 91
study, 2, 82, 111, 115, 118, 138, 140, 141, 147, 154, 156, 166, 186
style, 50
subset, 120
substance, 34, 93, 115
substitute, 47, 100, 174
success, 7, 28, 167
sugar, 70
suicide, 11
suitability, 137
summary, 62, 150
supervision, 21, 135, 170
supplement, 100
supplementation, 69
supply, 163
support, 5–7, 9–11, 14–19, 24, 28, 37–39, 41, 47, 59, 62, 63, 70, 79, 82, 83, 86, 89, 92–101, 107, 108, 117–120, 128–131, 135, 144, 147, 152, 153, 157, 160–164, 167, 170–176, 178–188
supporting, 15, 47, 58, 128, 135, 181
surge, 169
surrounding, 7–10, 29, 98, 100, 136–138, 142, 163, 172, 173, 187
susceptibility, 85, 139, 166
swimming, 73, 77, 81
symptom, 16, 18, 84, 117, 174, 187
symptomatology, 117
syndrome, 89
synthesis, 68, 70
system, 5, 6, 43, 49, 66, 85, 87, 93, 111, 112, 114, 118, 153, 159, 164, 175, 176, 179, 188

tai chi, 74
tailor, 18, 56, 117, 139, 146, 150, 165
tailoring, 17, 36, 145, 147–149, 166, 186, 187
talk, 42, 61, 107
target, 13, 112, 154, 180
teacher, 56
team, 81
teamwork, 188
technique, 24, 51, 57, 59, 60, 62, 63
technology, 94, 95, 100, 119, 120, 127, 128, 131, 146, 167, 169, 171, 172, 186
telecommunication, 120
telehealth, 120–124, 126, 159, 163, 169, 172, 179, 186, 188
telemedicine, 120–124, 126, 169
temperature, 85
tension, 54

term, 5, 23, 29, 85, 130, 133–136, 147, 170, 187
termination, 9
testing, 24, 147, 166, 167
text, 120, 169
theory, 39, 57
therapist, 18, 23, 24, 28, 45, 47, 48, 56, 86, 97
therapy, 4, 14, 17–19, 21, 23–29, 33, 39–48, 57, 59, 61, 93, 94, 101, 120, 126–128, 130–133, 135–138, 146, 159, 171, 185, 186
Thich Nhat Hanh, 56
thinking, 3, 23, 25, 27, 61, 63, 185
third, 87
thought, 17, 33, 61
time, 2, 6, 28, 48, 51, 56, 57, 74, 75, 79–82, 89, 90, 93, 97, 99, 101, 104–108, 127, 128, 130, 146, 167, 169–171, 175
tofu, 69
tone, 49
tool, 38, 42, 48, 57, 59, 61, 106, 127, 131, 175, 178, 185
torture, 4
toxicity, 135
track, 76, 128, 170
tracking, 83, 129, 170, 171
trainer, 82
training, 9, 21, 22, 24, 33, 35, 45, 48, 74, 76, 77, 79, 80, 128, 147, 149, 153, 160, 161, 163, 164, 170, 181–183
tranquility, 49, 55, 80
transformation, 13, 29, 41, 119
translation, 139
transmission, 112

transport, 68
transportation, 82, 93, 159, 169
trauma, 27, 42, 59, 62, 63, 100, 113, 139, 161, 185
travel, 159, 169
treatment, 1, 3–5, 8, 9, 11, 13–15, 17–20, 23, 24, 26–30, 34, 42, 44, 47, 58, 61, 62, 67–70, 75, 85, 86, 92, 93, 95, 114, 116–120, 127, 128, 130, 131, 133, 135–137, 139, 145–150, 159, 162–168, 170–174, 186, 187, 190
trial, 92
trigger, 26, 85, 126
trust, 19, 20, 28, 92, 97, 99, 130, 150
trusting, 28
turn, 3, 93
type, 76, 79, 92, 93

U.S., 137
ubiquity, 170
underpinning, 16
understanding, 2–5, 9, 10, 13–17, 19, 21, 44, 48, 49, 52, 56, 61, 67, 94–96, 99, 100, 105, 108, 111, 113, 114, 116, 130, 139–141, 145, 146, 148–151, 153, 154, 161, 173, 176, 180–182, 184–189, 191
unemployment, 11
unrest, 132
up, 55, 83, 85, 89, 118, 133, 140, 145, 170, 186
urbanization, 160
usability, 128
usage, 130

use, 13, 34, 39, 42, 45, 77, 90, 119, 127, 128, 131, 132, 134–138, 142, 147, 172, 178
user, 128, 130, 131, 172
utilization, 169, 180

validation, 93, 96–98, 100, 130, 173, 174
validity, 24, 127
value, 59, 97
variability, 129, 139
variation, 117
variety, 42, 139
vice, 2, 66, 118
video, 120, 169
vitamin, 68, 80
voice, 176
volunteering, 97
vulnerability, 96, 99

wake, 55, 85, 88, 89
walk, 74, 107
walking, 74, 82
way, 4, 29, 37, 48, 49, 83, 94, 114, 117, 119, 126, 133, 142, 145, 146, 169, 176, 182, 187
weakness, 154
week, 76, 80, 81
weight, 26
weightlifting, 74
welfare, 160, 179
well, 1–7, 11, 14–16, 20, 21, 27–32, 34, 38, 39, 41, 43, 48–56, 58, 62, 63, 66, 67, 69, 70, 79, 80, 83, 85–89, 92, 99, 101, 103, 104, 106–108, 114, 127–131, 133, 135–137, 139, 140, 142–145, 148, 150, 151, 153–155, 162, 164–166, 168–173, 175, 177–180, 182, 187, 188, 191
wellbeing, 5–8, 10, 13–19, 22, 36, 42, 45, 57, 58, 67, 70–76, 78–80, 92–101, 118, 119, 159–161, 178, 181, 183–187, 189
wellness, 5, 7, 51, 54, 79, 92, 96, 98, 101, 102, 104, 106, 107, 109, 143–145, 184, 185
whole, 68, 69, 143, 187
willingness, 28, 149
willpower, 108
wisdom, 29
witchcraft, 3, 20
withdrawal, 9
woman, 47, 75, 174
word, 49
work, 2, 7, 9, 17, 23, 27, 28, 39, 42, 48, 59, 74, 80, 82, 83, 92, 95, 107, 108, 120, 135, 159, 162, 169, 174, 176, 177, 182, 183
workforce, 9, 179
working, 16, 18, 84, 137, 138, 172, 182–184
workout, 75, 81
workplace, 7, 9, 11, 85
world, 13, 27, 95, 100, 126, 127, 159, 174, 175
worldview, 58
worsening, 84, 87, 187
worth, 4, 24, 28, 61, 93, 108
worthlessness, 25
writing, 57–63, 185

Index

year, 47, 75, 79

yoga, 17, 49–51, 54–56, 67, 75, 76, 80

zinc, 68–70, 72